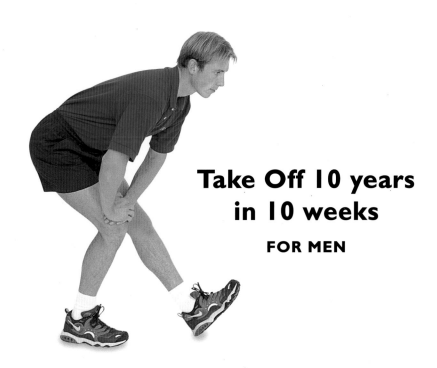

Take Off 10 years in 10 weeks

FOR MEN

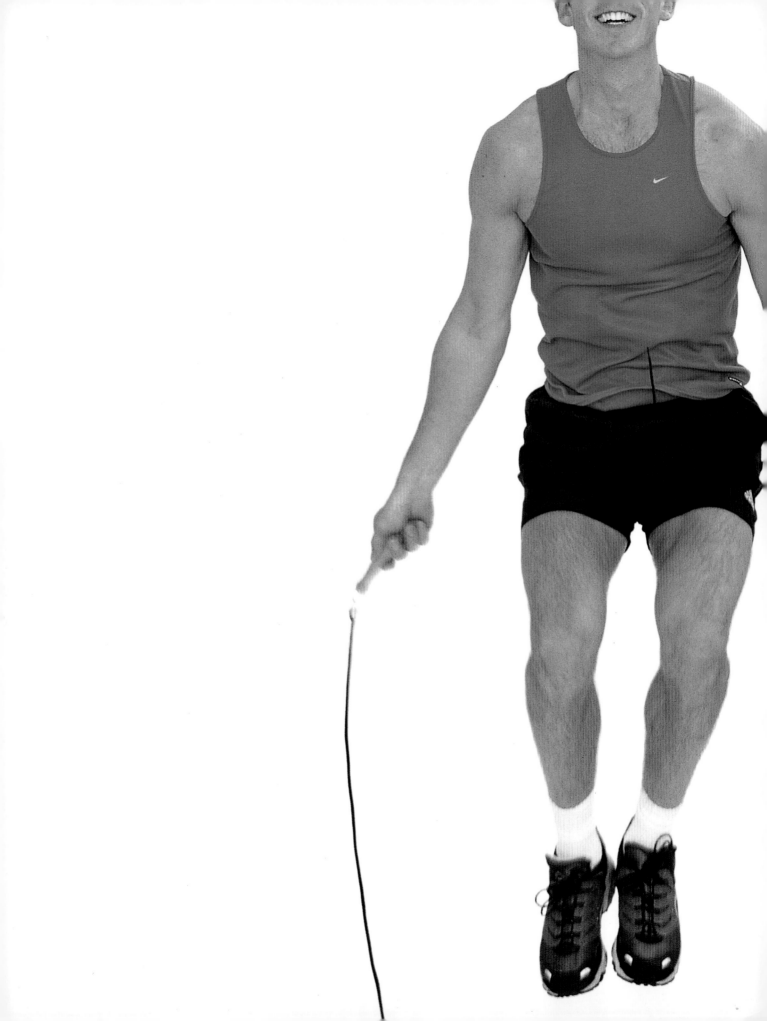

Take Off 10 years in 10 weeks

FOR MEN

JUDITH WILLS

WITH SPECIAL CONSULTANTS
Ceril Campbell, Phillip Hodson,
Rob Lander

SPECIAL PHOTOGRAPHY BY IAN HOOTON

Quadrille

TO TONY

Throughout this book both metric and imperial quantities are given. Use either all metric or all imperial, as the two are not necessarily interchangeable.

Publishing Director: Anne Furniss
Art Director: Mary Evans
Project Editor: Lewis Esson
Design: Mary Staples
Editorial Assistant: Rhian Bromage
Special Photography: Ian Hooton
Illustrations: Kathryn Adams
Production: Candida Jackson & Vincent Smith

SPECIAL CONSULTANTS
Sex & relationships: Phillip Hodson
Exercise: Rob Lander
Style: Ceril Campbell

First published in 1999 by
Quadrille Publishing Limited,
Alhambra House,
27–31 Charing Cross Road,
London WC2H OLS

Text © 1999 Judith Wills
Design & Layout © 1999 Quadrille Publishing Ltd

The rights of Judith Wills to be identified as the Author of this Work have been asserted by her in accordance with the Copyright, Design and Patents Act 1988.

Cataloguing in Publication Data: a catalogue record for this book is available from the British Library

ISBN   1 899988 39 4

Printed in Hong Kong

contents

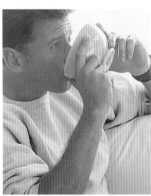

52

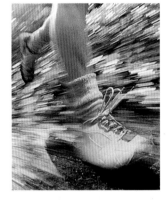

SECTION THREE

*getting
physical*

76

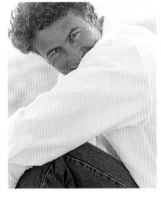

SECTION FOUR

*looking
good*

94

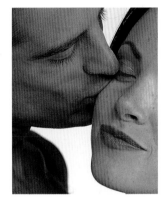

SECTION FIVE

*sex &
relationships*

108

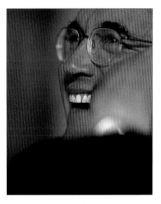

SECTION SIX

self

getting started

It's never too late.

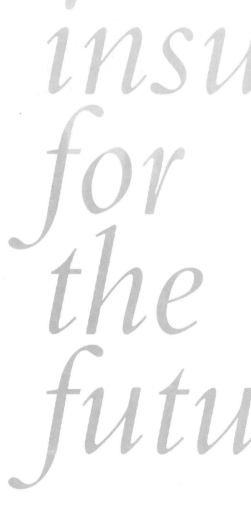

When I started writing the women's version of this title two years ago, I suspected that to feel younger, as well as look younger, was a priority for many women aged 40-plus. I was right – the book went on to become a best-seller worldwide.

Two years later, I have decided to do a '10-week' programme for men because, if anything, I feel that you males need it more! Let me throw some facts and figures at you. Men are 88% more likely than women to die from heart disease and 45% more likely to die from cancer. On average, middle-aged men are two stones overweight, and 90% suffer from stress, either at home, in sexual relationships or at work.

And yet men are less likely to look after themselves than women. About 60% don't take enough exercise to benefit their health – in mid-life and later, most manage only 30 minutes a week. Two-thirds drink too much alcohol and 40% work over 50 hours every week.

If you need this programme – you certainly want it, too. The male mid-life crisis is definitely alive and kicking. When we advertised for participants in the *London Evening Standard*, we had 400% more applicants than we had received for the female programme. Britain, it seems, is full of 40+ men going through what should be the 'best years' feeling just the opposite – 'past their prime', 'over the hill', unfit, unloved, unattractive, or just plain dissatisfied with their lives.

When we began the programme, I knew that we could make the men look better – good clothes, haircuts, and so on, can do wonders for anyone. What interested me perhaps most of all, however, was what difference we could make to their levels of fitness and health, which to me are the most important areas of concern for mid-life men.

As participant Chris Hampson, who has come fairly late to fatherhood, said,

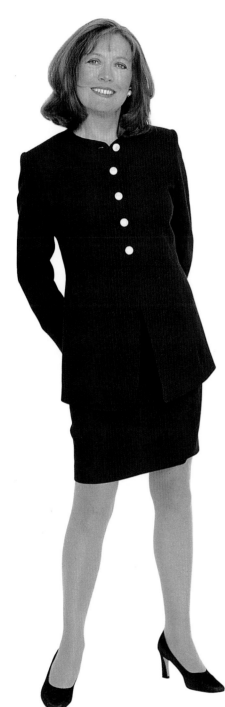

'Now I have children, I want to get my health and fitness back – it's insurance for the future. I owe it to my family.' Noel Ahearne, who married young and already has grandchildren, wants to be fit for them, too.

The fact is that physical fitness has a huge bearing on how well you feel both now, in everyday life, and in the future. The fact is that you don't have to 'lose it' as you get older – as all our men proved, you can improve your fitness profile 100% in as little as 10 weeks. This has the knock-on effect, as participants Chris Hall and Roger Douglas will tell you, of improving mid-life problems such as insomnia, anxiety, depression and weight gain.

To prove that the book lives up to its title, I devised an authoritative method of working out just how many years the men did shed within the 10 weeks. Before the programme we worked out their 'Real Age' – as opposed to their actual age in years – by scoring them in all areas of body, mind, health and lifestyle. You will be working out your own 'Real Age', too, before you begin. Then, 10 weeks later, the men did all the tests again and each had lost at least 10 years off his Real Age. I am sure you will too.

Apart from diet, fitness and style, we've also concentrated on your general quality of life, including your sex life, your relationships, your inner life and life at home and at work – or out of work.

I have enlisted the help of some of the top experts in the country to help you achieve your full potential – sex and relationship therapist Phillip Hodson, personal trainer Rob Lander, and stylist Ceril Campbell.

If you follow the 10-week programme, I hope that you will gain as much benefit as our four participants did – and keep the benefits going in the years ahead. Turn the page and meet the four men and, if you want some inspiration, turn to pages 132–5 to see them 10 weeks later. . .

FOUR TO WATCH

CHRIS HAMPSON

Chris, originally from Hull, used to be extremely active – cycling, going to the gym and playing football – but has found in recent years that his busy life has meant that keeping fit and slim slipped low down on the agenda.

He wrote to me saying, 'Life has been hectic in the last few years. I married Marcella in 1990, started my own business, had two children, and have just moved to a bigger property. Because of all this, I stopped cycling and found it hard to keep up the football and gym.

'The lack of exercise, coupled with sleepless nights, erratic mealtimes, snacking on the children's leftovers and eating and drinking as part of business, has meant that I'm now over 16 stone – at 6 feet 2 inches that's just too much.

'Having passed 40, and with dependants, I need to reconsider my lifestyle, my fitness and my health. But I need a kick-start to do it.'

CHRIS HALL

Chris was, to my mind, a typical 'middle-aged man', slipping – rather chaotically – into old age way before his time. He came to the programme feeling rather guilty about his lack of fitness. 'I belong to a gym, but only ever use the pool – can exercise machines ever be interesting? I occasionally play tennis in the summer and walk to work (about 20 minutes a day), but I don't feel this is enough. My weight has crept on, especially around the middle – at 5 feet 10 inches I'm over 13 stone. Too many snacks and sweet things between meals are probably to blame, too! I'm hoping you'll help me get back into shape.'

The other area in which Chris was keen to get help was fashion. 'I have no sense of style, and it would be interesting to have wardrobe advice.' We also thought that Chris was doing himself no favours with his haircut, moustache and sideburns, and hoped that as the weeks progressed he could be persuaded to go for a major change there!

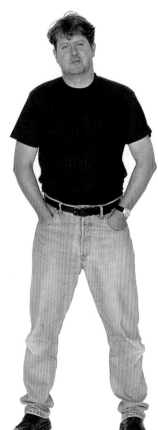

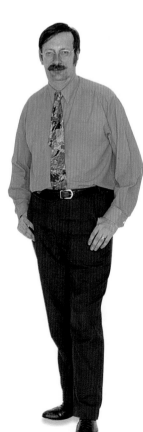

CHRIS

Actual Age: 41

Real Age: 44

Occupation: architect

Status: married with two children, aged 1 and 3

Lives: house in north London

CHRIS

Actual Age: 48

Real Age: 55

Occupation: litigation solicitor

Status: married with children, aged 13 and 15

Lives: Muswell Hill, London

MEET THE FOUR MEN WHO TESTED OUT OUR 10-WEEK PROGRAMME. THE PHOTOS OF THEM ON THIS PAGE ARE AS THEY ARRIVED TO MEET US BEFORE THE PROGRAMME STARTED. (THEIR REAL AGE PROFILES ARE DISCUSSED IN MORE DETAIL ON PAGES 18–19.) IF YOU WANT SOME INSPIRATION, TURN TO PAGES 132–5 AT THE BACK OF THE BOOK TO SEE HOW 10 WEEKS CHANGED THEM. THINK WHAT IT COULD DO FOR YOU. . .

NOEL AHEARNE

When Noel saw our advertisement he felt it was a 'last chance' to 'stop the rot'. With a basically sedentary lifestyle for many years – and a great social life, involving plenty of holidays, evenings out and weekends away – and 5 feet 10 inches in height, his waistline had burgeoned from a slim-line 32 inches in his young adulthood to a larger 38.

'I'd love to reshape my body,' he said, 'And my other aim is to get myself fitter, so that the family don't rib me when we go skiing this winter (as we do every year) about how unfit I am!' Noel smokes 20 a day and hopes to cut down during the programme.

I checked out his diet and found it was, to be frank, deplorable – lots of pastry and sweets, beer and little fruit or veg. I felt it would be in Noel's best interests, healthwise, to change his diet, especially considering he has high blood cholesterol, for which he has to take tablets.

We also thought Noel wasn't bringing out his personality in his clothing – jeans and yet more jeans – and stylist Ceril couldn't wait for him to shape up so she could 'get her hands on him' – fashionwise, of course!

ROGER DOUGLAS

When we met Roger he was in the process of splitting from a live-in partner and moving on his own to a new home in the Surrey countryside. He was also about to sign a contract for a new job, after being self-employed for 16 years. When he saw our ad for 'guinea pigs', he wrote in hoping we could help him feel, and look, more relaxed and less stressed. He also wanted to lose some weight off his 6-foot, 14 stone 10-pound frame and get back the fitness he'd lost over the years.

'I'm attempting to change my lifestyle (acquire one might be more accurate),' he said. 'I used to be pretty fit, but the combination of lazy diet, lack of exercise, lowering metabolic rate and fading will-power has taken its toll. I believe there's a link between physical and mental fitness, and I hope that physical fitness will help me cope with life's pressures.'

Roger looked smart, but rather dated, in the outfit he wore to meet us and his hair and glasses were not doing him any favours, so we felt he would enjoy the makeover to come at the end of the programme.

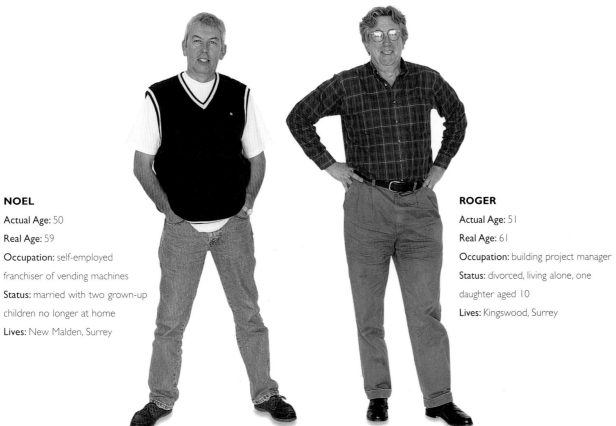

NOEL

Actual Age: 50

Real Age: 59

Occupation: self-employed franchiser of vending machines

Status: married with two grown-up children no longer at home

Lives: New Malden, Surrey

ROGER

Actual Age: 51

Real Age: 61

Occupation: building project manager

Status: divorced, living alone, one daughter aged 10

Lives: Kingswood, Surrey

BEFORE YOU BEGIN THE 10-WEEK PROGRAMME YOU NEED TO FIND OUT YOUR REAL AGE. IN ORDER TO DO SO, YOU MUST FIRST DO THE FOLLOWING THREE ASSESSMENTS – THE FAT FORMULA, HOW FIT ARE YOU? AND HEALTH CHECK, AND THEN WORK OUT YOUR REAL AGE AS SHOWN ON PAGES 16–17.

ASSESSMENT 1 – THE FAT FORMULA

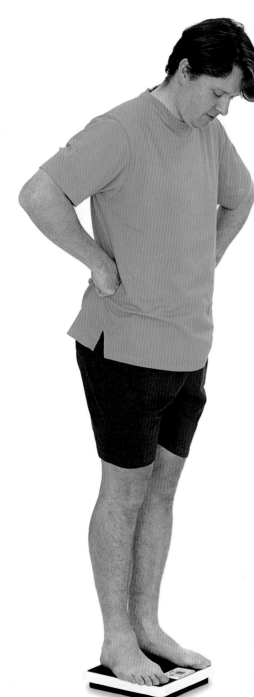

SURPLUS WEIGHT CAN ADD YEARS TO YOU, AND TAKE YEARS OFF YOUR LIFE-SPAN. IN FACT, FAT IS ONE OF THE MAJOR INFLUENCES ON **'YOUR REAL AGE'** (SEE PAGE 16). MOST OF US KNOW IF WE'RE A BIT OVER-WEIGHT, BUT JUST HOW OVERWEIGHT ARE YOU? FIND OUT HERE – AND ALSO FIND OUT HOW HEALTHY YOUR WAISTLINE IS.

There are two separate tests involved here – one for weight, the other for waist measurement. Simply do the two tests and add together your scores to obtain your own current Fat Formula.

The Body Mass Index

You need a calculator, pen, scales and measuring tape for your height.

❶ Weigh yourself without clothes. If necessary, convert to kilograms by dividing your weight in pounds by 2.2.

Your weight (kg) . . . .

❷ If necessary, convert your height in inches to metres by multiplying the inches by 0.025.

Your height (m) . . . .

❸ Square your height on the calculator (multiply it by itself).

Your height^2 . . . .

❹ Divide your weight in kilos by your height in metres squared to find your Body Mass Index.

$$BMI = \frac{\text{weight in kilos}}{\text{height in metres}^2}$$

Your BMI . . . .

THE GENERALLY ACCEPTED CLASSIFICATION FOR BMI IS:

Under 20	underweight – *poses health risk*
20-25	normal range of body weight
26-30	overweight – *health risk*
30+	obese – *very overweight – increased health risk*

In addition, recent research has shown that the ideal BMI for males – producing least risk of heart disease, ill health and early death – is around 22. We have produced a table of scores for BMIs taking all the current knowledge into consideration.

❺ So once you've worked out your BMI, check down the list here and find your current BMI SCORE.

Your BMI is	Your BMI Score is
Under 20	+2
20–21	0
21.1–22.5	-2
22.6–25	0
25.1–29.5	+2
29.6–35	+3
Over 35	+4

WRITE YOUR BMI SCORE HERE

Waist circumference

Your waist measurement is another important indicator of your health, risk factors for illness and shortened life-span – and real age. Various methods have been devised for assessing your relative risk – waist-to-hip ratios, waist-to-height ratios, etc., but it has been found that the simplest test of all is virtually as accurate as anything else – you just measure your waist.

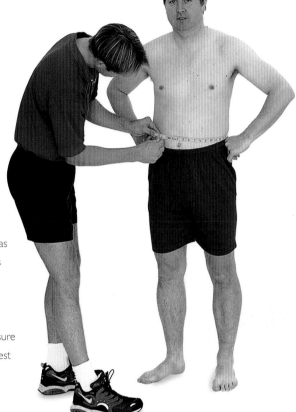

❶ With no clothes on, take a tape measure and measure your waist around its smallest part. Don't pull tight, so that the skin is puckered – the tape should be snug, neither loose nor tight.

Waist Circumference . . . .

❷ Now check the list below to find the score for your waist measurement.ment.

Waist Circumference	Health Risk	Waist Circumference Score
Under 90 cm (35.5 in)	Low	-2
90–93 cm (35.5–36.5 in)	Moderate	0
94–101 cm (37–40 in)	Increased	+2
Over 101 cm (40 in)	High	+4

WRITE YOUR WAIST CIRCUMFERENCE SCORE HERE . . . .

*Now add together your **BMI score** and your **Waist Circumference** score. The result is your **Fat Formula** score.*

YOUR FAT FORMULA SCORE IS . . . .
Keep this safe – you will need it to complete Assessment 4, your Real Age Assessment.

ASSESSMENT 2 - HOW FIT ARE YOU?

LACK OF FITNESS IS PERHAPS THE GREATEST NEGATIVE INFLUENCE ON YOUR REAL AGE. FITNESS IS FOUR-PRONGED – STAMINA, STRENGTH, FLEXIBILITY AND POSTURE – AND THE TESTS ON THIS PAGE ASSESS ALL FOUR AREAS.

● Take the tests as soon as is convenient, wearing suitable clothing – shorts and a T-shirt are ideal, plus a comfortable pair of training shoes.

● You will also need a pen.

● If you have any history of heart trouble, you should check with your doctor before beginning these tests and if you can't complete any test without pain, stop and see your doctor for advice.

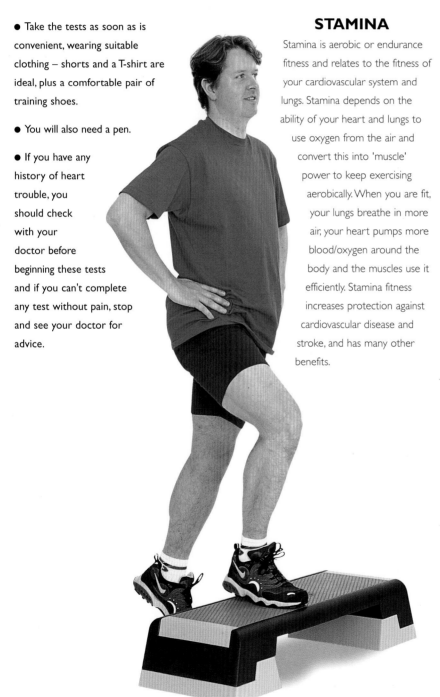

STAMINA

Stamina is aerobic or endurance fitness and relates to the fitness of your cardiovascular system and lungs. Stamina depends on the ability of your heart and lungs to use oxygen from the air and convert this into 'muscle' power to keep exercising aerobically. When you are fit, your lungs breathe in more air, your heart pumps more blood/oxygen around the body and the muscles use it efficiently. Stamina fitness increases protection against cardiovascular disease and stroke, and has many other benefits.

The Step Test

To carry out this test you will need a step, stair or similar, about 30 cm (12 inches) high in a convenient place.

❶ Step up and down on it for 3 minutes exactly. (Technique – step up with right foot, up with left foot, down with right foot, down with left foot, to complete one step. Then step up leading with the left foot, then right, down left, down right. And so on. Stand near the base of the step, not too far away.)

❷ Immediately the 3 minutes are up, check down the chart here to find the perceived exertion level that most closely matches your own:

Exertion level	Your score
1 You found the exercise easy and feel fine.	☐ -2
2 You found the exercise moderately easy and you are slightly out of breath.	☐ -2
3 You found the exercise moderately hard and are fairly out of breath.	☐ 0
4 You found the exercise hard and are very out of breath.	☐ +1
5 You found the exercise very hard and are extremely out of breath.	☐ +2
6 You found the exercise too hard and couldn't complete the 3 minutes.	☐ +3

RECORD YOUR SCORE HERE ☐

FLEXIBILITY

Body stiffness, lack of flexibility in the joints and a narrow range of movement are all associated with ageing. Keeping supple and flexible is an important part of keeping young. The test here measures the flexibility of both lower back and hamstrings.

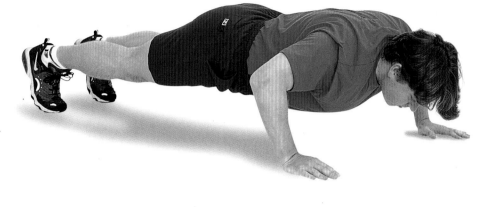

The Sit and Reach Test

Do not do this test when your body is cold – if necessary, warm up first with a walk, marching on the spot or other aerobic activity.

Sit on a mat on the floor with your legs straight out in front of you, hip-width apart, feet flexed (toes pointing towards the ceiling), arms at your sides, lower back unslumped, shoulders relaxed. Stretch out your fingers towards the toes. How far can you go and hold for a count of 3?

Reach		Your score
1 No further than mid-lower leg		+2
2 Around ankles		+1
3 To toes but no further		0
4 Beyond toes		-2

RECORD YOUR SCORE HERE

STRENGTH

Strength is how much force you can exert to push, pull, lift and so on. Muscular strength declines rapidly with age if it isn't maintained with weight-bearing exercise. Upper body strength is a good indication of all-over strength and the following test is the best indicator of upper body strength.

The Press-up Test

Kneel on a floor mat on all fours. Keeping spine strong, stomach tucked in and head and neck in alignment with your back, move feet backwards and lift knees off the floor until body weight is supported by arms and toes. Smoothly lower body to 4 inches (10 cm) from floor, then raise it again, using your arms' strength and keeping the spine strong as before. This counts as one press-up.

Continue until you can't do any more (your arm muscles will begin to shake). Rest.

Number of press-ups		Your score
Less than 6		+2
7–13		+1
14–20		0
21–30		-1
Over 30		-2

RECORD YOUR SCORE HERE

POSTURE

Poor posture is a real give-away of age and can add years on to any man. Check your posture here.

Stand with your back against a wall. Can you stand with back of head, shoulders, tail-bone and heels all touching the wall at the same time?

Posture test		Your score
Yes		-2
No		+2

RECORD YOUR SCORE HERE

YOUR SCORES

Stamina

Flexibility

Strength

Posture

TOTAL FITNESS ASSESSMENT SCORE *

*Add up any plusses first, then subtract the minusses.
Keep this score safe – you will need it to complete Assessment 4, your Real Age Assessment.

ASSESSMENT 3 – HEALTH CHECK

YOUR GENERAL STATE OF HEALTH AFFECTS NOT ONLY YOUR CHANCES OF LIVING A LONG AND HEALTHY LIFE BUT ALSO HOW YOU FEEL NOW – YOUR ZEST AND ENERGY LEVELS. IF BOTH ARE LOW, YOUR REAL AGE WILL APPEAR HIGHER. SO DO THIS HEALTH CHECK NOW AND SEE HOW YOU GET ON.

NOTE: If you have a high 'plus' score in any one or more of these health check sections, see your doctor or appropriate practitioner and make sure to carry out the parts of this 10-week programme that are most likely to help you.

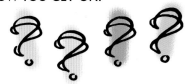

ALCOHOL

How many alcohol units do you drink a week? I unit equals I glass of wine, a half-pint of beer, cider or lager, or I single measure of spirits.

Consumption in units	40+	28+	15-28	7-14	None
Your score	+2	+1	0	-1	0

Your **Alcohol** score . . . . . ☐

SMOKING

How many cigarettes do you smoke a day?

Cigarettes per day	40+	20+	1–20	None
Your score	+3	+2	+1	0

Your **Smoking** score . . . . . ☐

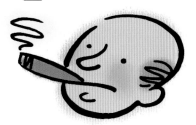

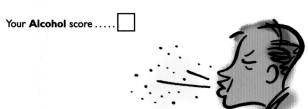

ILLNESSES AND COMPLAINTS

How often do you suffer from the following? Circle your score on each line.

	Often	Sometimes	Rarely/never
Colds	+2	+1	0
Flu	+2	+1	0
Chest infections	+2	+1	0
Skin/eye infections	+2	+1	0
Cold sores	+2	+1	0
Mouth ulcers	+2	+1	0
Bleeding gums	+2	+1	0
Constipation	+2	+1	0
Heartburn	+2	+1	0
Backache	+2	+1	0
General aches, pains, stiffness	+2	+1	0

Add on 2 points for any chronic diagnosed medical condition you suffer – e.g. diabetes, high blood pressure.

Add up your total and check here for final complaints score:

Your total	Your final complaints score
+15 or more	+2
+8 to +14	+1
0 to +7	0

Your **Complaints** score . . . . . ☐

DIET

How often do you eat any of the following? Circle your score on each line.

	Often	Sometimes	Rarely/never
Fruit	-1	0	+1
Vegetables	-1	0	+1
Fish	-1	0	+1
Whole-grain cereals	-1	0	+1
Pulses	-1	0	+1
Full-cream milk	+1	0	-1
Full-fat dairy produce	+1	0	-1
Red meat	+1	0	-1
Desserts/cakes/biscuits	+1	0	-1
Chocolate and sweets	+1	0	-1

Add up your total and check here for final diet score:

Your total	Your final diet score
+6 to +10	+2
+1 to +5	+1
-5 to 0	0
-10 to -6	-2

Your **Diet** score . . . . . ☐

MIND AND LIFESTYLE

Check your scores for each of the following questions.

1. *Using a watch to time yourself, can you memorize the opening two sentences of the first paragraph on the back cover of this book, and say them out loud in:*

☐ I minute or less? score -1

☐ 2 minutes or less? score 0

☐ over 2 minutes or not at all? score +1

2. *Using a watch to time yourself, can you recite the alphabet backwards without slipping up in:*

☐ 30 seconds or less? score -1

☐ I minute or less? score 0

☐ over I minute or not at all? - score +1

3. *Without sleeping pills, do you wake in the morning feeling refreshed?*

☐ Yes score -1   ☐ Sometimes score 0   ☐ Rarely score +1

4. *Do you take a walk (or similar) in the fresh air every day?*

☐ Yes score -1   ☐ No score +1

5. *Do you take time out every day to relax and do something enjoyable?*

☐ Yes score -1   ☐ No score +1

6. *Do you have sex regularly?*

☐ Yes score -2   ☐ No score +2

7. *Do you frequently work long hours?*

☐ Yes score +1   ☐ No score -1

8. *Do you regularly have to drive long distances/in rush hour?*

☐ Yes score +1   ☐ No score -1

9. *Would you say that you have good energy levels?:*

☐ Most often score -1 ☐ Sometimes score 0 ☐ Rarely score +1

10 *Do you feel tired after adequate hours of sleep?*

☐ Rarely score -1   ☐ Sometimes score 0   ☐ Often score +1

Add up your total and check here for final mind and lifestyle score:

Your total	+6 to +11	+1 to +5	0	-1 to -5	-6 to -11
Your final score:	+4	+2	0	-2	-4

Your **Mind and Lifestyle** score . . . . . ☐

STRESS

Circle your answer on each line.

How often do you suffer from the following emotions?

	Often	Sometimes	Rarely/never
Upset at small things	+1	0	-1
Angry or resentful	+1	0	-1
Isolated or lonely	+1	0	-1
Inadequate or useless	+1	0	-1
Anxious, nervous	+1	0	-1
Depressed	+1	0	-1

Add up your total and check here for final stress score:

Your total	+4 to +6	+1 to +3	0	-1 to -3	-4 to -6
Your final score:	+2	+1	0	-1	-2

Your **Stress** score . . . . . ☐

OUTER YOU

Score 1 for each Yes answer: Yes

1. Are your teeth all your own? ☐
2. Are your teeth in good condition? ☐
3. Are the whites of your eyes bright and clear? ☐
4. Is your skin a healthy colour? ☐
5. Is your skin smooth and pleasant in appearance? ☐
6. Is your hair plentiful? ☐
7. Is your hair shiny and healthy? ☐
8. Do people ever take you for younger than you really are? ☐

Your total	5-8	2-4	Under 2
Your final score	2	-1	0

Your **Outer You** score . . . . . ☐

To find your total Health Check score:

Add up your scores in each of sections – alcohol, smoking, diet, illnesses, mind and lifestyle, stress and outer you. (You may like to add up all the plus scores first, then add up the minus scores and subtract them from the plus score to reach your final total.)

Your total HEALTH CHECK SCORE is . . . . ☐

Keep this score safe – you will need it to complete Assessment 4, your Real Age Assessment.

ASSESSMENT 4 – YOUR REAL AGE

BY ADDING TOGETHER YOUR SCORES FOR ALL THREE PREVIOUS ASSESSMENTS, AND FINALLY ADDING ON YOUR ACTUAL AGE, YOU WILL ARRIVE AT WHAT I HAVE CALLED YOUR 'REAL AGE'. THIS IS ONE TEST THAT NO MAN IN HIS MIDDLE YEARS – OR OLDER – SHOULD MISS.

How old are you? Your Real Age may be considerably different from your actual age. Real Age takes into account all the physical, lifestyle and mental factors that go to help make you feel old. If you feel 'old before your time', you may take this test and discover that your real age is perhaps 20 years older than your actual age. You may also, of course, find that your real age turns out actually to be younger than your calendar years. In which case – you've probably bought the wrong book!

Don't be too shocked by the results – if the calendar says you're 45 and your Real Age turns out to be 75, for instance, then all is not lost! The test is a light-hearted look at how you may have been taking your life and your health for granted.

Motivation

However, a Real Age score that is much above your current actual age means that, without doubt, there is plenty you can – and should – do to lower your Real Age, and increase your health and well-being. We all have a natural tendency to 'let ourselves go' as we get older and it is this process that you can reverse – with the right kind of help and motivation.

As the Real Age test only includes those factors about which you can do something positive – fitness, diet,

lifestyle, and so on – it is a great motivation to take up the challenge this programme presents.

Your score is also subjective – it's up to you to answer the questions as honestly as you can, but the test can never be properly scientific. (Your Real Age assessment doesn't take account of how up-to-date or otherwise you are in the style department – Section 4 of the book can also help take years off the way you look.)

The idea of this book is to help you lower your Real Age over the course of 10 weeks – and, as you will discover by reading about our participants Noel, Roger and the two Chrises, it really is possible to take at least 10 years off your Real Age assessment in the 10 weeks. Your aim is to get your Real Age down to at least your actual age, and it is possible to reduce it even lower. If, for instance, your Real Age and your actual age turn out to be the same – you can still use the book to help you. Why be average for your age when you could be amazing?

You will need to know your Real Age to get the most out of the book, and to participate in Section 3 – Getting Physical.

Growing Younger

If you continue with all the many healthier habits that you will learn in the programme, over the months ahead – and, hopefully, for the rest of your life – your Real Age will gradually reduce even more, thus ensuring that as you get older . . . you really get younger!

You will be re-doing the assessments once or twice during the 10-week programme to check how you are progressing. After that, I suggest you repeat the process every three months or so, and seeing your Real Age drop will give you all the incentive you need to carry on with a healthier lifestyle, and a lifestyle that is more comfortable for you.

A low Real Age is a good indicator of how long you will live and how healthy, fit and full of zest you will feel, and how young you will look and seem to others, throughout your life.

Note: The Real Age assessments don't work for men younger than 40 years or over the age of 80.

To find out your REAL AGE:

❶ Fill in your scores from the 3 assessments on the previous pages in the table (right).

❷ Total them up.

❸ Add (or subtract) the total to (from) your actual age in calendar years.

example

Your **FAT FORMULA** score was	+4
your **FITNESS** score was	+2
your **HEALTH CHECK** score was	-1
giving you a total **ASSESSMENT** score of	+5
Your **ACTUAL AGE** is	46

Add together your **ASSESSMENT** score and your **ACTUAL AGE**

and your **REAL AGE** is	51

YOUR SCORE

Assessment 1 (Fat Formula) score	☐
Assessment 2 (Fitness) score	☐
Assessment 3 (Health) score	☐
TOTAL ASSESSMENT SCORE	☐
YOUR ACTUAL AGE	☐
YOUR REAL AGE	☐

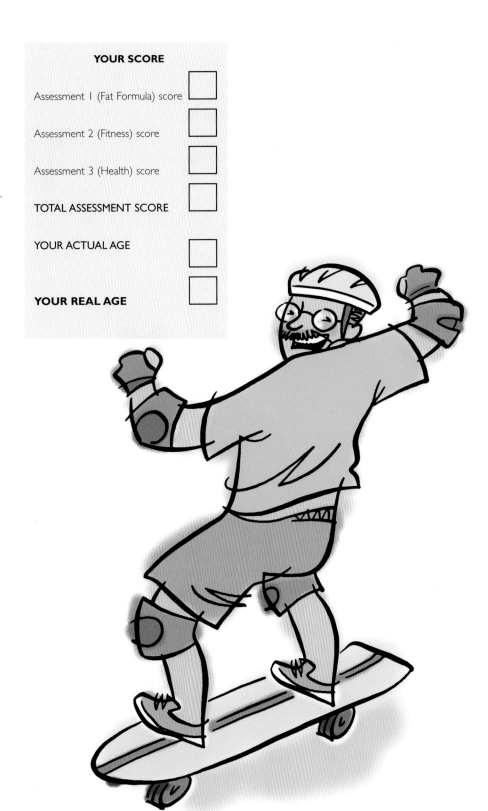

ASSESSING OUR PARTICIPANTS

CHRIS HAMPSON

Chris is in very good general health, with quite low stress levels despite his hectic life. He is also quite strong and his posture is good. However, his stamina level is poor for a man of his age – probably partly because he is carrying too much weight. His Body Mass Index (BMI) is over 30 and therefore his weight is categorized as a health risk. We measured his body fat percentage at 22.5% – the normal range for a man is 14–20%. Much of this fat sits around his belly and his waist circumference places him at high risk of health problems. We need to slim him down, reduce his total body-fat percentage and improve his stamina – the three goals that Chris himself has prioritized.

CHRIS HALL

Chris has a typical 'middle-aged man' shape, with weak upper body – small chest, weak arms and shoulders – and poor posture, as well as a 'pot belly', and a poor score for both BMI and waist circumference. His all-round fitness is fairly poor, although his overall health isn't too bad. He has a very high body-fat percentage for a man, at 27.8%, and a low percentage of lean (muscle mass) at 74.8% (the average male should have from 80–86% lean). We will be working on all areas of Chris's fitness and helping him to lose body fat, with a sensible eating programme. Chris also suffers from bouts of mild depression and anxiety, and Rob has assured Chris that regular exercise will also help him to feel better mentally.

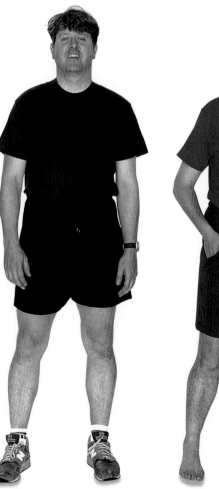

CHRIS

Height: 6 ft 1 in (1.83 m)

Weight: 16 st 2 lb (102.7 kg)

Chest: 43 in (1.07 m)

Hips: 43 in (1.07 m)

Body Mass Index: 30.9

Waist Circumference: 40.5 in (1.01 m)

FAT FORMULA SCORE: +7

Stamina (step test): Level 5

Strength: achieved 22 press-ups

Flexibility: achieved Level 3

Posture: passed the test

FITNESS SCORE: -1

HEALTH CHECK SCORE: -3

Total Score for all Assessments: +3

Actual age: 41

REAL AGE: 44

CHRIS

Height: 5 ft 10 in (1.75 m)

Weight: 13 st 9 lb (86.8 kg)

Chest: 39.5 in (99 cm)

Hips: 42 in (1.05 m)

Body Mass Index: 28.4

Waist circumference: 39 in (98 cm)

FAT FORMULA SCORE: +4

Stamina (step test): Level 4

Strength: achieved 10 press-ups

Flexibility: achieved Level 2

Posture: failed the test

FITNESS SCORE: +5

HEALTH CHECK SCORE: -2

Total Score for all Assessments: +7

Actual age: 48

REAL AGE: 55

WE ASSESSED ALL FOUR OF OUR PARTICIPANTS USING THE FAT FORMULA, THE FITNESS ASSESSMENT AND THE HEALTH ASSESSMENT, TO COME UP WITH THEIR CURRENT PROFILES AND THEIR OWN REAL AGES.

NOEL AHEARNE

Noel is only very slightly overweight, but with most of that surplus concentrated around his belly – giving him an 'increased risk' score for his waist circumference profile. Exercise, and cutting back a little on his alcohol intake, rather than a strict diet, should decrease this without trouble. Noel also has poor posture in his upper body, which gives the impression of a poor body shape. Strength and flexibility work will help to reshape him and increase his body tone. We will also concentrate on improving his stamina levels – Noel likes to go skiing with his family and is fed up of being ribbed over his lack of fitness on the slopes. Noel's health isn't bad, but he does smoke and he is aiming to cut down over the weeks ahead – Rob has explained to him that cigarettes and exercise just don't mix.

ROGER DOUGLAS

Roger looks quite young for his age, but when Rob carried out the fitness tests we realized that, in fact, he was very unfit and with a BMI and waist circumference both likely to give him an increased risk of heart disease in later life. His chest and hips are well proportioned, though, and we felt that, given the right exercise programme coupled with healthy eating, he would shape up very well indeed! One of the 'old before his time' signs was his lack of flexibility ('I can't even bend over to tie my shoelaces!' he complained) and general stiffness and aches and pains. Rob assured him that plenty of work on suppleness would help there. Roger also fell down on his lifestyle score and stress levels, so we will be working with him to find ways to help him relax.

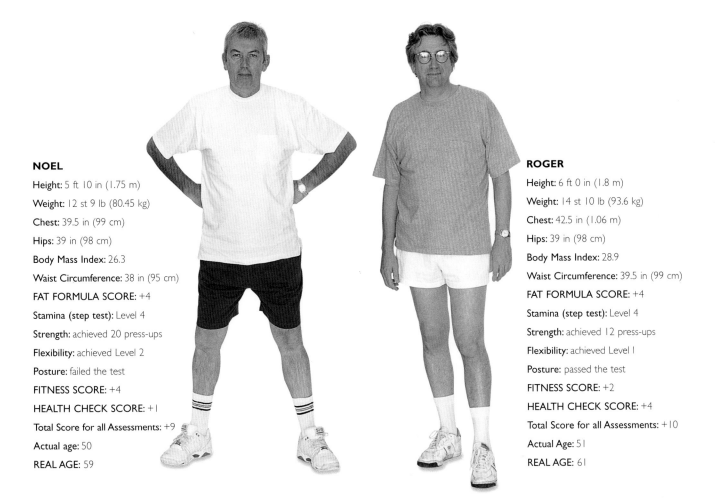

NOEL

Height: 5 ft 10 in (1.75 m)

Weight: 12 st 9 lb (80.45 kg)

Chest: 39.5 in (99 cm)

Hips: 39 in (98 cm)

Body Mass Index: 26.3

Waist Circumference: 38 in (95 cm)

FAT FORMULA SCORE: +4

Stamina (step test): Level 4

Strength: achieved 20 press-ups

Flexibility: achieved Level 2

Posture: failed the test

FITNESS SCORE: +4

HEALTH CHECK SCORE: +1

Total Score for all Assessments: +9

Actual age: 50

REAL AGE: 59

ROGER

Height: 6 ft 0 in (1.8 m)

Weight: 14 st 10 lb (93.6 kg)

Chest: 42.5 in (1.06 m)

Hips: 39 in (98 cm)

Body Mass Index: 28.9

Waist Circumference: 39.5 in (99 cm)

FAT FORMULA SCORE: +4

Stamina (step test): Level 4

Strength: achieved 12 press-ups

Flexibility: achieved Level 1

Posture: passed the test

FITNESS SCORE: +2

HEALTH CHECK SCORE: +4

Total Score for all Assessments: +10

Actual Age: 51

REAL AGE: 61

food & drink

There is a great deal of truth in the old saying that 'you are what you eat'.

you are what you eat

A child can't grow and thrive without the right nutrients, and an adult can't survive and flourish without them either. As we grow older, the right diet is even more important in offering protection against most of the wear and tear of the years.

To give you a few examples: your muscle mass won't remain adequate unless you eat sufficient protein; your skin will get dry and old before its time if you don't eat sufficient nutrients and drink plenty of water; your bones may suffer from mineral depletion if you eat a diet that's short in the right balance of minerals or too high in protein; your joints may become inflexible earlier than normal without sufficient essential oils; your body-fat content will be too high if you consume too many calories, or too low if you don't consume enough – and so on.

Good nutrition also affects your general well-being in other ways – your energy levels, stress levels, sleep patterns, your teeth and gums, your eyesight, sex life and even your mood. It also offers protection against the major diseases of our time – cardiovascular disease and cancer – and against a myriad of the other ills of middle-age, such as digestive disorders, diabetes and obesity.

You will be finding out more about how to eat for all areas of your well-being throughout the book. This section is concerned with the basics of good nutrition and with weight control.

Good nutrition is a two-sided affair. One, it is about cutting down on the things that are less 'good for you' (this is the first aspect most people consider when they look at their eating habits). Two, probably even more important, it is about getting enough of the things that *are* 'good for you'.

So, firstly in this section, we sort out the nutritional facts from the fiction and give you all the info you need in a nutshell. Then we go on to provide four different eating plans to suit everyone, plus a questionnaire to help you decide which one is right for you.

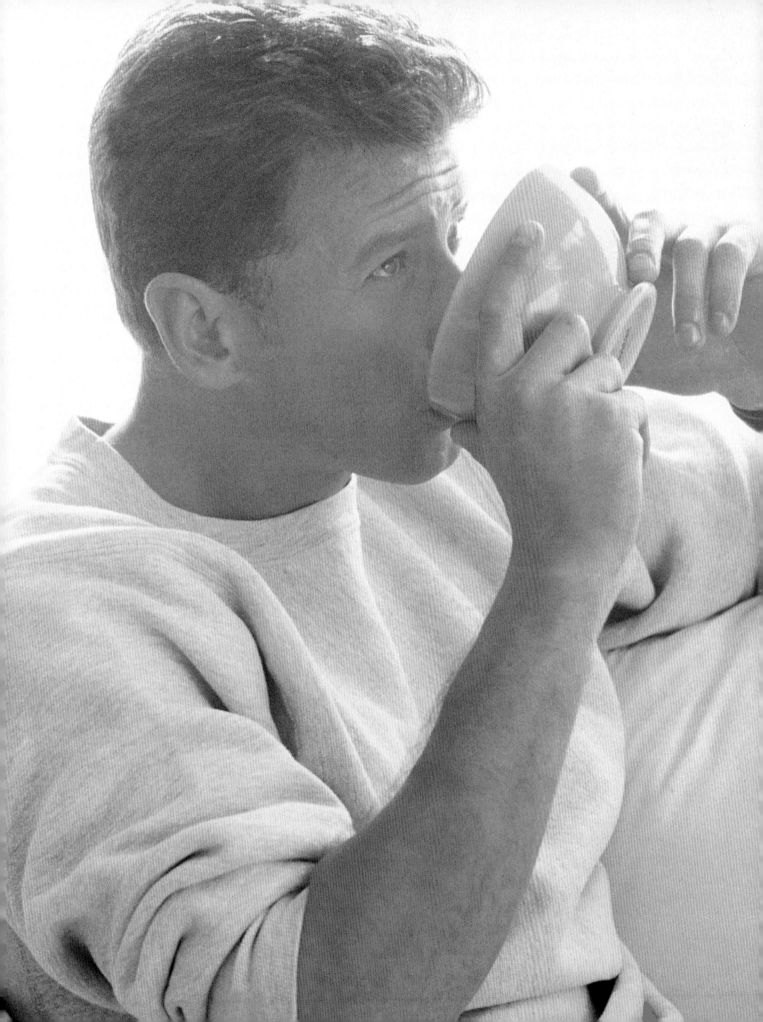

TEN FOOD MYTHS EXPLODED

IF YOU STILL THINK THAT BAKED BEANS ARE BAD FOR YOU, OR THAT ALL MEN NEED MEAT – READ ON!

MYTH

Men need a lot of meat in their diets

Meat is a good source of protein – along with various other foods. such as milk, cheese, eggs and lentils. In order to make muscle, and keep it, everyone needs to eat enough protein – the 'building blocks' of lean tissue (under which category muscle comes).

If you take the 'average' man compared with the 'average' female of the same height, the male will usually have more lean tissue (80–84% of total body matter) than the woman (at 72–78%) – while women have a higher natural body fat composition, at 22–28% compared to men's 16–20%. Therefore, in official guidelines, adult men's requirements for protein are slightly higher than females, at 40–55 grams per day or 0.75g of protein per day per kilo of your body weight – representing no more than about 10% of a total day's calorie intake.

Most people eat much MORE protein than this. Some estimates put the protein content of the average western male diet at 25%+ – a level which may be detrimental to health, as too much dietary protein (especially animal protein) can decrease bone mass and may also be linked with increased blood pressure.

A professional bodybuilder may need extra protein, but for the average moderately active man of 35+, large steaks, huge plates of roast meat or big bacon-and-sausage fry-ups are not only unnecessary but nutritionally way out of date. For one thing, meat (and dairy pro-duce) can be a source of unwanted saturated fat (see Fat on page 26) as well as calories.

If you're exercising hard and feel the need for protein, rather than eating more meat you would probably be better off with a bowl of lentil soup or a plate of stir-fried tofu. Vegetable protein sources like these tend to be much lower in fat and calories and higher in goodies such as fibre. The fact is that many men would be much healthier for increasing their intake of starchy carbohydrate foods, like bread, potatoes and grains, and fruits and vegetables, rather than worrying so much about protein. Yes, meat is a good source of iron, but men need *less* iron in the diet than women do – and, anyway, lentils are a terrific source of iron, along with many other non-meat foods!

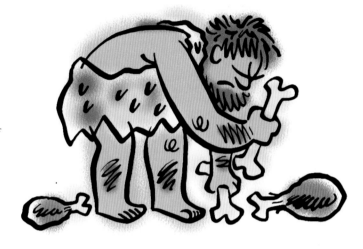

MYTH

A fat-free diet is the healthiest of all

There is no such thing, really, as a fat-free diet that is healthy. About the only foods that contain no fat at all are sugars, some herbs and spices, and some drinks such as colas, diet drinks, squashes, water and alcohol. All fruits and vegetables have fat in them, ranging from quite a lot (as in avocados or coconuts), moderate amounts (as in Brussels sprouts and sweetcorn) through to hardly any (as in limes or blackcurrants). Even black tea and coffee have tiny amounts of fat in them. So to follow a fat-free diet would be very hard – a healthy fat-free diet is impossible.

The fact is that we all do need some fat in our diets. We especially need plant fats – or oils. Foods such as cereals, nuts, seeds, pulses and vegetables contain unsaturated fats (see Fat, page 26) which are essential for a healthy body and good skin, hair, and so on. Oily fish contains a type of fat (the omega-3 oils EPA and DHA) which is particularly good for maintaining a healthy circulation and can help prevent strokes and heart disease. Olive oil is high in monounsaturated fats (as are avocados and many nuts) which are also 'good for you'.

So don't feel guilty about eating some high-fat foods in your diet – even on the low-fat eating programme in this book you will find reasonable amounts of these 'good-for-you' fats.

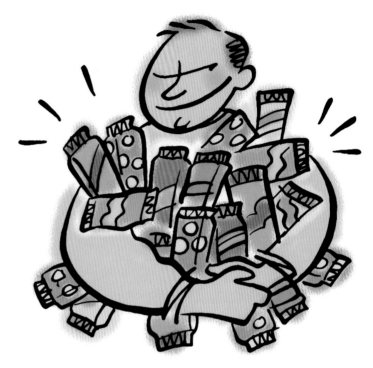

MYTH 3

Carbohydrate and protein shouldn't be mixed at the same meal

Fans of the system called 'food combining' (the Hay system), which seems particularly popular with men, will say this – the idea being that the digestive system can't cope with protein (meat, fish, dairy, etc.) and carbohydrate (bread, potatoes, pasta, etc.) eaten at the same time, and therefore it gets all sluggish and confused and clogged up, and we gain weight and have trouble losing it.

This is all nonsense! One, our bodies have been coping happily with mixed meals for years. Two, the theory (for which there isn't a shred of scientific evidence) falls down when you consider that some of our healthiest foods contain both protein and carbohydrate in the same package – e.g. all pulses.

The reason people lose weight when they begin food combining is that because the diet is so restrictive they are taking in many less calories than usual. It's as simple as that.

For food combining fans, I have come up with my Carb-3 plan (pages 40–3) – a much gentler diet that is easier to follow, and produces equally good weight-loss effects!

MYTH 4

Starchy foods are fattening

Starchy foods – such as bread, potatoes, pasta and rice – are part of the carbohydrate group of foods, which also encompasses sugars. Many of the earliest slimming diets of the 60s and 70s attempted to cut out starch from the diet altogether for easier weight control.

Looked at logically, this can't be ideal. The calorie-providing nutrients in food are protein, fat and carbohydrate. Both protein and carbohydrate contain around 4 calories per gram; while fat contains 9 calories per gram. The only other nutrient which provides calories is alcohol, at 7 calories a gram. Therefore, logically, it is fat and alcohol that one should mainly cut down on to save calories. As we've seen in Myth 1, most people eat too much protein, so that should come next if we need to cut down further. For health reasons, too, it is important to get enough starch in the diet. Cereal foods, pulses, fruit and root veg provide fibre, vitamins and minerals, and are essential for a healthy gut and colon. Therefore, if you're going to cut carbs – make it sugar first.

MYTH 5

Certain foods, such as sugar and chocolate, are addictive and should be avoided

There is no scientific proof that sugar, as such, is addictive in the true sense – i.e., you can't get physically hooked on sugary foods as you can on, say, alcohol or tobacco or hard drugs.

However, people who eat a lot of sugar may experience something akin to withdrawal symptoms if they suddenly cut sugar out of their diet, particularly if the diet is nutritionally poor in other respects. This is normally because the blood sugar levels will drop drastically if the 'sweet toother's' normal intake is stopped, resulting in feelings such as light-headedness, dizziness, fatigue – and sometimes cravings for something sweet!

Chocolate is only addictive in so far as it contains sugar and caffeine, which is a stimulant, but the caffeine content in most chocolate is so small that it wouldn't produce true addiction.

Both sugar and chocolate can be eaten in moderation as part of an overall healthy diet – to prevent the craving for more, it is always best to use them as part of a meal rather than on their own as a snack, when blood sugar levels are more likely to go haywire.

MYTH

Middle-aged spread is normal and impossible to shift

Our metabolic rate (the rate at which we burn calories) does slow down gradually after the age of about 30–35. It has been estimated that this represents about 50 calories less a day for every 5 years. For example, if you are 45 you may need 100 calories less a day than you did aged 35 in order to maintain the same weight; at 55 you'd need 200 calories less; at 65, 300 calories less.

To give you an idea of how much that is, one average slice of bread and butter would be about 100 calories, and so would one large banana or half a pint of beer.

So, if one doesn't take steps to prevent it, this slowing metabolism will result in steady weight gain over the years. Also, for both men and women, the extra fat tends to accumulate around the stomach/waist – the typical middle-aged 'spread'.

The figures are, however, based partly on the known fact that for most people, lean tissue (muscle mass) diminishes as we get older, and lean tissue is 'metabolically active'; so, if we lose muscle, we lose some of our ability to burn calories. Some of this muscle decrease is inevitable, especially as we get to 60+, but the decline *can* be halted, or even reversed, in middle age IF we take more exercise, particularly weight-bearing exercise, like walking, or strength exercise like gym work. Exercise also burns calories in other ways, not just by increasing muscle mass.

A sensible diet, cutting down a little on the less nutritious items in our diet, such as alcohol and saturated fat, will also result in saving the necessary few calories to avoid weight gain. But the best idea of all is to combine the two – watching what you eat a little, and exercising a little. This is not only the best combination for your weight in middle age, but also for your health.

Therefore, middle-aged spread (if that is taken to mean putting on weight as we get older) could be called 'normal' – but inevitable it certainly isn't! Some experts believe that a small weight gain of up to a stone on one's youthful weight is desirable, as underweight can lead to health problems such as loss of bone mass and insufficient intake of vitamins and minerals, leading to deficiencies. More than this, however, is probably not a good idea – especially for men.

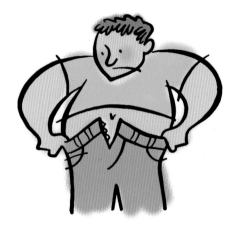

MYTH

Fasting is a good way to clear out the system

The occasional one-day fast won't do you any harm, except perhaps to give you a headache and make you feel irritable, but fasting for weeks at a time on nothing but water isn't healthy or practical for most of us. Far from 'clearing out the system', it can actually lead to constipation and digestive problems, and can release 'free radicals' into the system which may actually increase the risk of heart disease or cancers.

The best type of 'clear out' is simply one where you avoid 'junk foods' and eat a wide range of really healthy, natural foods, such as those that form the basis of the Detox Programme on pages 46–9.

MYTH

Dieting is bad for the brain

One piece of research has shown that people on diets appear to be less mentally alert and 'on the ball' than those who aren't dieting. Most experts believe that the explanation for this result is simply that people on diets (many of which are of the 'crash' type – too low in calories and likely to produce hunger and deprivation) spend a lot of time thinking about food, thinking about their weight problems and so on, and have less time and mental/emotional energy to spend on their work.

There is little evidence that a sensible slimming programme will produce this effect or that properly constructed diets may affect the brain because they are too low in nutrients. In fact, there is evidence to show that too much food – particularly refined carbohydrates like white bread – can slow down the brain and lead to poor performance and fatigue.

MYTH
Dieting slows your metabolism and makes you fat

Another old tale that is not true. The only proper scientific research carried out on this subject was at the world-famous Dunn Nutrition Centre in Cambridge. The research, led by one of our top obesity research scientists, proved that even people who repeatedly yo-yo diet end up with a metabolic rate the same as someone (of the same age, weight, etc.) who hasn't dieted. If dieting made you fat, how come people deprived of food long-term (say during wars or famines) aren't fat? If you go on a sensible weight-loss diet, reach a sensible target weight and then eat a normal diet (not going back to the diet that made you fat in the first place), then it is quite possible to maintain your new, slimmer weight.

This, I think, is where this myth began. For it is quite true that your metabolic rate will be less when you weigh, say, 12 stones, than it was when you weighed, say, 16 stones. The larger the body, the more work it has to do to maintain itself. Work equals calories burnt. Therefore, as you slim down, your metabolic rate naturally reduces, because there is less work to do, but when you weigh 12 stones after dieting, your metabolic rate *won't* be different from a 12-stone person who has never dieted. You only get fat if you eat more than you need to maintain your current weight!

MYTH
Men need more calories than women

Not necessarily. It depends on your height, age, activity levels and so on. The 'average' man, according to the DoH, needs around 2,550 calories a day up to the age of 60, then his needs drop to 2,380 and then after 65 further to 2,330. This is around 500 calories a day more than the 'average' woman.

However, if you happen to be on the short side, aged 60 and fairly inactive, and you are married to a woman who is on the tall side, aged 30 and fairly active, it is a fair bet that she will need more calories a day than you! If you're eating more than her, you're probably getting fatter and wondering why, and she isn't getting fatter, and you're saying it isn't fair . . .

You can alter the balance by getting more exercise (see Myth 6), but sadly there is not a lot you can do about your height or age!

If you are both the same height and age and do the same amount of activity, then you will probably need to eat more than her as she has less muscle (maybe! – see Myth 1).

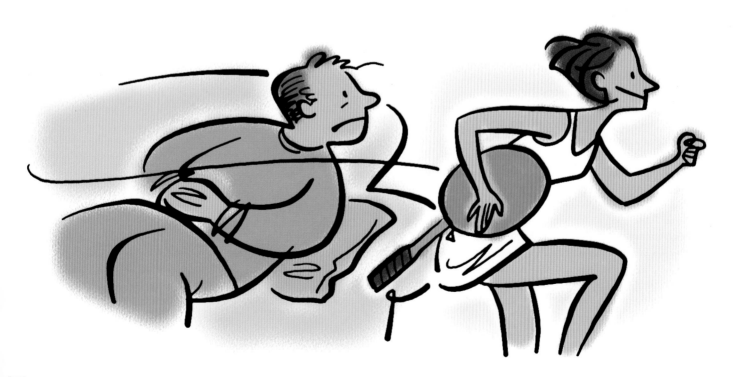

Nutrition in a Nutshell

YOU NEED TO KNOW WHY YOU NEED TO EAT A GOOD HEALTHY, VARIED DIET OTHERWISE YOU'LL NEVER STICK TO IT. HERE YOU'LL FIND A QUICK REFERENCE TO ALL THE MOST IMPORTANT NUTRIENTS: WHAT THEY ARE, WHAT THEY DO AND WHERE TO FIND THEM.

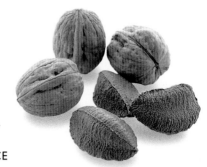

MAJOR *ENERGY-GIVING* NUTRIENTS

FAT

What it is: made up mainly of fatty acids, important in the diet for energy (either converted directly into energy during, for example, prolonged exercise or stored in the body as body fat and converted when needed). Some fats, called essential fatty acids, are vital in the food we eat, albeit in small quantities.

Different types of fat are implicated in our health in different ways.
Saturated fat is found in largest quantities in dairy produce and meats, lard, suet and many manufactured foods, such as chocolate and pastries. It is the first type of fat to cut down on as it is linked with increased risk of cardiovascular disease and other possible ills.
Trans fat, also known as hydrogenated fat, has a similar effect on the body as saturated fat – it is not a natural fat, but is polyunsaturated fat hardened by chemical processes and is present in many commercial foods, including margarines, biscuits, cakes and others.
Polyunsaturated fat are usually liquid at room temperature. This group contains the essential fatty acids (see above). which we need in small regular quantities for good health. Good sources are sunflower, corn, sesame and walnut oil, Brazil nuts, all oily fish (mackerel, salmon, tuna, trout, herring, sardines), nuts and seeds. Polyunsaturated fats can help lower blood cholesterol – but too much may be harmful. They are best kept cool, eaten raw and fresh, as cooking or incorrect storage can oxidize them, producing free radicals – minute particles which, if produced in excess in the body, may be responsible for ageing, increased risk of heart disease and cancers.
Monounsaturated fat is another good form of fat which can help to maintain a healthy heart by lowering blood cholesterol levels and may also help prevent cancers. Olive, rapeseed and groundnut oils are excellent sources, as are avocados, some nuts and seeds.

CARBOHYDRATE

What it is: there are two types of carbohydrate in the diet, starch and sugar. The starchy carbohydrates, found in greatest quantities in plant foods, such as cereals, pulses, root vegetables, are called 'complex carbohydrates' and are an essential part of the diet for good health – about 50% of our daily calories should come from these foods. Complex carbohydrates are also present in all fruits and vegetables but, because of the high water content of most fruit and veg, the carbohydrate content is low.

When complex carbohydrates are refined (as in white bread, white rice, white pasta), some of the essential goodness of the raw ingredients is removed (mainly fibre and vitamins/minerals); so, as a general rule, it is better to eat the whole grains, etc., rather than highly refined produce. However, refined carbohydrates such as bread, rice and pasta can form part of a healthy diet.

Sugars form about 40% of the carbohydrate that we eat – either added to foods and drinks by ourselves or in ready-to-consume form, such as in soft drinks, cakes, biscuits, pastries and so on. Sugar isn't essential to our health – containing no nutrients except calories – and so, if overweight, it is a good item to cut down on.

PROTEIN

What it is: formed from amino acids, 22 of which are used in the body to build muscle and for other body functions.

Eight of these amino acids need to be provided in our diet and these are called 'essential amino acids'. Meat, fish, eggs and dairy produce, as well as soya beans, contain all eight essential amino acids and are therefore called 'complete proteins' (they used to be called 'first-class proteins'), but today it is recognized that a good balanced healthy diet will include many of the vegetable sources of protein, such as lentils, chickpeas, baked beans. If taken as part of a varied diet, high in complex carbohydrates and nuts and seeds, these will be perfectly adequate for good health and forming muscle mass.

Some animal protein foods are also high in saturated fat (see left) and should be limited when on a weight-reducing diet – these are fatty cuts of meat, whole milk, whole yoghurt, and many cheeses, including Cheddar, cream cheese and Stilton. Eggs are a medium-fat food. Oily fish are high in fat, but shouldn't be limited as they contain healthy types of fat (see left).

Good lower-fat protein foods include lean fillet of pork, poultry (skin removed), game (including venison, pheasant, wild duck, rabbit), white fish, shellfish, pulses, skimmed milk, semi-skimmed milk, fromage frais and low-fat yoghurt.

MICRONUTRIENTS

VITAMINS

What they are: there are eleven organic micronutrients essential for health and needed in the diet as our bodies can't manufacture them. You are unlikely to be going short of some, while it is harder to ensure adequate intake of others, listed here.

Vitamin C an antioxidant vitamin (helping to neutralize the free radicals that can cause disease and ageing, see opposite). Water-soluble, so can't be stored in the body; needed every day. Needs increase if you smoke, drink, are ill or under stress.
Good sources most fresh or frozen fruits and vegetables.

Beta-carotene converted to vitamin A in the body, beta-carotene is another antioxidant.
Good sources found in orange-, red- and yellow-fleshed fruits and vegetables, especially carrots, sweet potatoes, squash, cantaloupe melon, red peppers, tomatoes and leafy greens.

Vitamin E another antioxidant vitamin and also important in maintaining a healthy immune system and protection against cancer. Vital for healthy skin, hair, nails. Any junk diet is likely to be short of this vitamin.
Good sources include wheat germ, sunflower and safflower oils, nuts, seeds, and other oils.

B vitamin group a group of six vitamins needed every day as they are water-soluble and can't be stored in the body. Needs increase if you drink alcohol, smoke or are under stress. Depleted in the diet through storage, heat, cooking and light.
Good sources a varied healthy diet, including lean meat, poultry, vegetables, whole grains, nuts, low-fat dairy produce, oily fish and seeds, will ensure adequate intake of all six.

MINERALS

What they are: inorganic substances, 15 of which are needed in small-to-very-small amounts in the diet for a variety of functions. A shortfall of many of these minerals is unlikely; those listed here are those most likely to be deficient in the diets of Western males.

Calcium needed, along with vitamin D (from sunlight and margarine) and essential fatty acids, for strong bones; deficiency of calcium has also been linked with heart disease.
Good sources dairy produce (cottage cheese isn't a particularly good source), dark leafy greens, nuts and seeds, white bread, fish.

Iron deficiency can cause anaemia, though this is more common in women.
Good sources red meat, lentils, dark leafy greens, offal, fortified break-fast cereals, eggs, dried apricots, brown rice. (Vitamin C aids absorption; tea drinking can hinder absorption.)

Zinc essential for fertility and reproductive system, good skin and immune system, among other things. Smoking and alcohol may reduce zinc levels.
Good sources include lean meat, whole-grain cereals, nuts, seeds and pulses.

Selenium another antioxidant, helping to protect against ageing, heart disease and cancers. Strong likelihood of lack in many diets.
Best source Brazil nuts, also lentils, other nuts, fish, whole-grains. Levels vary according to where food is produced, as soil levels vary considerably.

Magnesium helps energy levels and nerves. Also important for a healthy heart. Alcohol intake can affect absorption.
Good sources include nuts, seeds, soya, liquorice.

Potassium essential, particularly if you have a high-salt diet. Helps to regulate blood pressure and many body functions.
Good sources found in good quantities in most fresh fruits and vegetables, dried fruits, nuts and pulses.

SODIUM

Also a mineral but, in the Western world, is the one dietary mineral that many of us get too much of and that we may need to cut down on. Sodium is the main component of common salt, and a high-sodium diet has been linked with high blood pressure and heart disease. A diet containing many highly processed foods will be high in salt; a natural diet of fresh fruits and vegetables (cooked with very little or no added salt), whole-grains, and so on, will be much lower in sodium, although even fresh vegetables do contain sodium.
High-sodium foods include: salt, stock cubes, packet soups, bacon, ham, deli meats, ketchup, pickles, processed cheese, corn flakes, savoury snacks. Check labels for sodium content.
We should aim to eat no more than 4g of salt a day (1,600mg sodium).

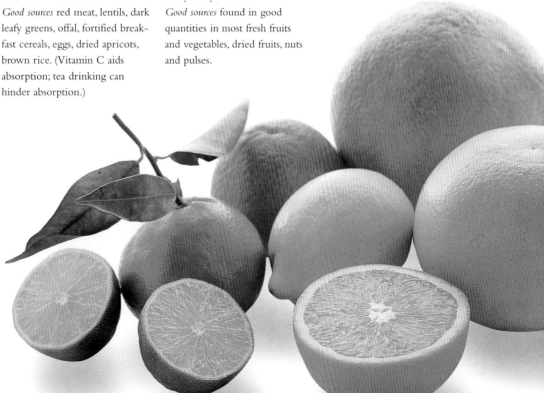

YOU AND ALCOHOL

ALTHOUGH A LITTLE DRINK CAN BE GOOD FOR YOU, HEAVY DRINKING IS A CONTRIBUTORY FACTOR TOWARDS MANY ILLS, INCLUDING SOME CANCERS, HEART DISEASE, LIVER PROBLEMS, AND OBESITY. PERHAPS IT IS TIME TO TAKE A LOOK AT YOUR OWN ALCOHOL INTAKE.

The group of people in the UK with the highest rate of alcohol intake are middle-aged men, with over 50% drinking more than the safe levels recommended by the Department of Health.

What is a healthy amount of alcohol?

You don't have to drink alcohol to be healthy, so the obvious answer is 'no alcohol at all'. In fact, most research shows that a small amount of alcohol – particularly red wine or the darker beers like stout – can be good for men in their middle and later years. One or two glasses a day can help to minimize the risk of heart disease by altering the balance of the 'good' and 'bad' cholesterols in the blood. However, one or two glasses are all that it takes.

What is the most I can drink and stay healthy?

Safe levels for men have been set at 3–4 units of alcohol a day. One unit equals one-sixth of a bottle of table wine (8% alcohol by volume); one single measure of spirits or half a pint of beer, cider or lager. Saving up units for one or two binges a week is unsafe.

How does alcohol affect my REAL AGE?

As we've seen, one or two glasses a day may actually help keep your heart healthy and you will probably feel and look fine on that amount as a regular

thing. But heavy drinking can affect your weight. Alcohol is quite high in calories at 7 calories per gram. An average double Scotch or glass of wine or half of beer will set you back about 100 calories. One pound of body fat is equivalent to 3,500 calories consumed – so you can see how a few drinks a night (say, 500 calories' worth) could easily put a pound a week on your waistline.

It also affects your mental powers – your memory, your concentration, your agility – and your physical powers – your coordination, your potency, your libido.

Your facial features may change, with the typical drinker's red nose, florid cheeks, jowls, yellow-tinged eye whites, and so on. An overworked liver (which processes the alcohol in your body) can result in you looking and feeling permanently off-colour and run down. Alcohol depletes various nutrients in the body and is a depressant.

How can I cut down?

Once you realize the health implications of heavy drinking you may find that you can cut down quite easily. You could go 'cold turkey' (giving up completely straight away), which may have you feeling uneasy for the first few days, but within a week you will be fine. Alternatively, you could cut down gradually, say a glass less every night until you are down to just one or two glasses; or

you could choose lower-alcohol drinks, or water down your wine, for example. Some people find they don't miss wine if they drink grape juice.

There are many ways to do it but whichever you choose you may need a prop, and the best prop is to keep busy and find other ways to enjoy yourself – or relax, the reason many men drink too much. (By the way, alcohol will relax you at first, but long-term it IS a depressant and can increase your stress levels by upsetting your sleep patterns and affecting your ability to work well.)

Other tips are to eat a very healthy diet, high in complex carbohydrates (see previous page) and fresh fruits and vegetables, with enough low-fat protein. Such a diet will help to keep your blood sugar levels even and will help prevent cravings for something sweet – often mistaken for the craving for alcohol.

But what if I can't cut down?

If you can't cut alcohol down or out and are drinking more than 3 or so units a day, then get professional counselling, see your doctor or join Alcoholics Anonymous, where some of the greatest men in the world have learnt how to stay dry.

If you're just drinking a little, then you can carry on doing so as a small amount of alcohol is okay on all but the Detox and Energize Eating Programmes.

CHEAT'S GUIDE TO WEIGHT LOSS

NOTHING ADDS YEARS ON YOU LIKE SURPLUS WEIGHT. YOU NEED TO GET RID OF IT AND

SHED SEVERAL REAL AGE YEARS IN THE PROCESS. LOSING WEIGHT ISN'T HARD – IF YOU KNOW

HOW TO AVOID THE DREADED PITFALLS OF HUNGER, BOREDOM AND DEPRIVATION.

(EATING OUT, AND ALL ITS PITFALLS, ARE DISCUSSED ON PAGES 50–51.)

THE 'H' WORD

Will you be hungry on your diet? In the first couple of days you may feel a little hungry – or, at least, think that you are. After that, however, once you have the right mind-set and your stomach has given up expecting its usual high-fat feast several times a day, plus extras, you shouldn't feel hungry at all.

Whichever of the four plans you choose, there is plenty to eat in terms of weight of food, volume of food and amount on the plate. Because you are going to be eating in a slightly different way from normal, however, you may find these tips useful in overcoming your fear of the dreaded hunger:
● Eat all you're allowed on your eating programme. Skipping meals is a recipe for a Snickers binge.
● Eat frequently. That means don't let more than 2½–3 hours elapse before eating something during waking hours. You do this by having a breakfast, a lunch and an evening meal, with two small snacks – one between breakfast and lunch and the other between lunch and evening. If you have to have your evening meal very early (say at 6 p.m. and don't go to bed until 11 p.m.), then you may be better off having your second snack in the evening.
● Learn to tell real hunger from fake hunger. Sometimes you may think you are hungry when you are not. Boredom, frustration and stress can sometimes manifest themselves as 'I

must have something to eat'. Also be wary of other people offering you food you don't really want. You'll say yes before you realize it.

It will help you control your food intake sensibly if you keep a food diary for a week or two, writing down what you ate, and why. Put a cross through all the food you ate when you didn't really need it and you'll see how many calories and how much fat you could have saved.
● Real hunger? Feed it. The technical reason for initial hunger pangs is the stomach signalling the brain that it is empty. You may also get hunger signals from the brain, however, if your blood sugar levels are low, which is why the meals in your eating programme will contain plenty of the foods that have a low or medium Glycaemic Index, meaning that they take longer to be converted into glucose and keep your blood sugar levels more constant.
● If a true hunger-pang really does attack you, have a small piece of a high-protein, low-fat food that also contains a little carbohydrate, such as a small pot of low-fat yoghurt. The carbohydrate will be absorbed first, getting your blood sugars back to normal, and then the protein will take longer to be absorbed, keeping you feeling full until the next meal. Chocolate just isn't necessary.

BOREDOM

'Boring diet food' is a bit of a cliché now, isn't it? Weight loss conjures

up pictures of cardboardy, airy crispbreads, dabs of tasteless cottage cheese, bits of limp lettuce and, if you're lucky, a cup of hot water with a slice of lemon in it. If that's your idea of how to lose weight, I expect you're still fat.

I need do no more than suggest you look through the meal suggestions contained in the following four eating programmes.

You will see, with some relief I hope, that you can choose from a wide range of foods on all four of my plans. One plan will appeal to you more than the others (see the quiz overleaf). If you pick the one that appeals most, you are unlikely to be bored.

The point of modern weight-loss programmes is that you *can* stick with

them. The old 'yo-yo' diets happened because you could only be 'good' for a few days in a row without throwing in the towel and bingeing on cheese or chips.

I am lucky in that I find most of the so-called 'healthy' foods delicious and tempting, especially when enlivened with spices, herbs, and all the kinds of non-fattening seasonings that you can get these days that can transform the plainest of dishes. Things like vegetables and fruits in season, nuts, grains and fish I can happily live on without complaining, as long as I also get regular small doses of white wine and roast lamb.

I hope to prove to you that eating right can be enjoyable and tasty and that you need be neither deprived nor bored.

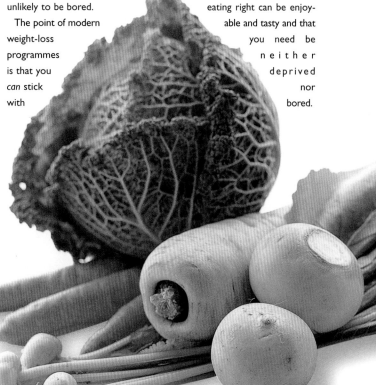

THE EATING PROGRAMMES

PREFERENCE QUIZ

- *Tick the yes or no boxes in each column.*
- *Add up the 'yesses' at the end of each column.*
- *Then read your preferred diet choice in the Results panel.*

Column 1

	yes	no
1. I have tried many diets in the past without success.	☐	☐
2. I like an ordinary, varied diet.	☐	☐
3. I often eat with the family/others.	☐	☐
4. I am often reliant on other people preparing my food.	☐	☐
5. I don't really want to give up many foods.	☐	☐
6. I don't like the idea of a set, strict regime.	☐	☐
7. I have a sweet tooth.	☐	☐
8. I tend to eat what is in front of me and not go back for more.	☐	☐
9. I don't find between-meal snacking much of a problem.	☐	☐
10. I agree with *'a little of what you fancy does you good'.*	☐	☐

Column 2

	yes	no
1. I want an easy and relaxed eating plan.	☐	☐
2. I prefer savoury tastes to sweet ones.	☐	☐
3. I don't want to count calories.	☐	☐
4. I enjoy bread, potatoes, rice, pasta.	☐	☐
5. I have a big appetite and dread feeling hungry.	☐	☐
6. I enjoy a little alcohol.	☐	☐
7. I enjoy seafood, fish, game, poultry.	☐	☐
8. I am willing to cut down on red meat.	☐	☐
9. I am willing to cut down on cheese.	☐	☐
10. I want my new diet to be as healthy as possible.	☐	☐

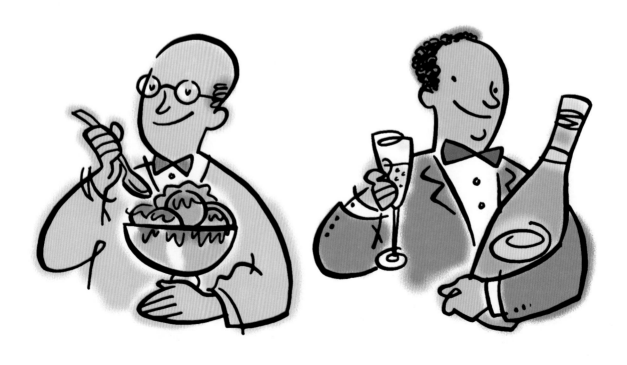

YOU NEED TO CHOOSE ONE OF THE FOLLOWING FOUR EATING PROGRAMMES TO HELP YOU LOSE WEIGHT (IF NECESSARY) ON THE 10-WEEK PROGRAMME. TO HELP YOU DECIDE WHICH IS RIGHT FOR YOU, COMPLETE THIS LITTLE QUESTIONNAIRE AND THEN CHECK YOUR RESULTS.

Column 3

yes no

1. I feel like something different to try.

2. I want an easy diet with no weighing or measuring.

3. I can live without a cheese sandwich.

4. I don't want to give up meat, but I could eat it without potatoes.

5. I like bread, potatoes, rice, pasta.

6. I enjoy vegetables and fruit.

7. I am prepared to plan ahead.

8. I don't need to buy take-away lunches/meals very often.

9. I think of myself as open-minded.

10. I don't often have to eat with other people.

Column 4

yes no

1. I feel like a complete overhaul, nutritionally.

2. I often worry about my intake of sugar, salt, caffeine, additives.

3. I have easy access to good food stores.

4. I am organized and determined.

5. I have adequate time to spend reorganizing my diet.

6. I am happy to cut certain things out of my diet completely.

7. I often feel guilty about my current eating/drinking habits.

8. I do really want to change.

9. I need to lose weight.

10. I enjoy fruits, vegetables, salad – or, at least, would like to develop a taste for them.

RESULTS

● Add up your 'yesses'. Which column did you get most in?

● Check here for your preferred diet:

Most in Column 1:
Your preferred programme is Portion Power, beginning on the next page.

Most in Column 2:
Your preferred programme is the Fat Control programme, beginning on page 36.

Most in Column 3:
Your preferred programme is Carb-3, beginning on page 40.

Most in Column 4:
Your preferred programme is Detox, beginning on page 46.

● *Begin your chosen programme straight away.*

NOTE: *If your yes scores tied in two or more columns, look at your equally preferred programmes and, on reading them, see which you prefer. You can swap later on in the 10 weeks if you want to.*

PORTION POWER

IF YOU'RE NO GOOD AT SPECIAL DIETS AND WANT TO CUT CALORIES, SAVE FAT AND LOSE WEIGHT WITHOUT BASICALLY CHANGING YOUR EATING HABITS, THE PORTION POWER PROGRAMME IS PROBABLY THE ONE FOR YOU.

In the main, the Portion Power programme involves simply reducing the size of the portions of all high-calorie foods on your plate, from between one-third and a half, maintaining portion sizes of moderate-calorie foods, and increasing portion sizes of low-calorie foods.

I have worked out that an average overweight man will save between 600 and 900 calories a day by using this method – enough to lose 1–2 pounds a week without doing anything else at all!

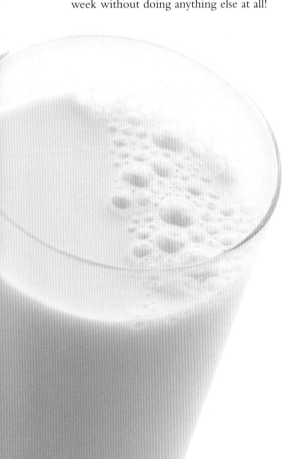

All you do is follow the simple illustrated instructions overleaf for all lunches and main meals. You choose a breakfast from the LOW-FAT breakfasts that appear on page 37. And you also have some Unlimited foods, a daily milk and fruit allowance and a weekly Treat allowance, all of which are listed on the right. Items which don't appear in any of these lists should be avoided (e.g. cakes, biscuits, puddings) unless having them as part of your weekly Treat units.

Try to space your meals out evenly during the day, vary your meal choices as much as possible and *do* remember to eat plenty of the Unlimited vegetables and salads with each and every lunch and main meal. If you don't, you may feel hungry and may not be getting all the nutrients you need for good health and good looks.

INSTRUCTIONS

Unlimiteds

Eats

All vegetables of all kinds, except potatoes and sweet potatoes, to be lightly boiled, steamed, microwaved, baked or raw. Eat plenty of leafy greens, raw salad items and peas and beans, onions, tomatoes, lettuce, water-cress, carrots. Eat what you enjoy! Vegetables can be fresh or frozen or, occasionally, canned.

Condiments

Lemon and lime juice, fresh or dried herbs and spices, tomato purée, passata, Worcestershire sauce, light soy sauce, vinegar, low-fat stock cubes, chilled ready-made stock.

Drinks

Water – drink up to 2.25 litres (4 pints) a day; mineral water; weak tea or coffee (with milk from allowance or black preferably without sugar); low-calorie diet drinks and squashes and mixers. Water is the drink of preference – for good skin, good digestive system and proper hydration. If exercising regularly, you need water. Tea, coffee and cola drinks do not count towards your day's fluid intake.

Milk allowance

Up to 200 ml (7 fl oz) semi-skimmed milk a day for use in tea and coffee, or as a drink on its own.

Fruit allowance

2 pieces of fresh fruit a day (or 2 average portions, in the case of things like berries, pineapple).

Weekly treat allowance

Every week you are allowed 14 units of 'treats' (see overleaf). It is best to spread your Treat units evenly over the week, not using them all up in one or two days, especially where alcohol is concerned.

EXAMPLE

An example of how you can save nearly 1,000 calories a day on your diet just by following the Portion Power principles:

				SAVING	
LUNCH-TIME	3 large pork sausages as part of a sausage-and-mash lunch	420 calories	*Swap* to 3 chipolata sausages (keeping the mash)	210 calories.	
			To help fill you up: Add 3 tablespoons of baked beans for 45 extra calories, plus any unlimited vegetables if liked	45 calories	SAVING on lunch 165 calories
MAIN MEAL	275 g (10 oz) steak	500 calories	*Reduce* to 175 g (6 oz) steak	300 calories	
	225 g (8 oz) chips	615 calories	*Reduce* to 125 g (4½ oz) chips	341 calories	
	1 rounded tablespoon mayonnaise on side salad	140 calories	*Reduce* to 1 level dessertspoon (2 level teaspoons)	70 calories	
			To fill you up: Add large servings of peas or sweetcorn and broccoli	about 80 calories	SAVING 464 calories
	to follow 60 g (2½ oz) Cheddar cheese	250 calories	*to follow* *Reduce* to 25g (1 oz) cheese	104 calories.	SAVING 116 calories
			Add small piece of fruit to fill up the plate	30 calories	SAVING on main meal 580 calories
					Total calories saved on the two meals = 745

● Such a saving represents over 5,000 calories in a week, which would convert to about 1½ pounds of weight lost.

● If you choose to SWAP some high-fat items for lower-fat items, you could have even more to eat while making similar savings.

For example, if you swapped 125 g (4½ oz) chips (341 calories) for 200 g (7 oz) new potatoes (144 calories) you would have an extra 75 g (2¾ oz) of potato to eat for nearly 200 calories less, thus losing weight a little more quickly again.

● Just follow the Portion Power principles on your favourite foods, listed overleaf – and you can lose weight as easily as that.

THE SIMPLE RULES OF PORTION POWER

EACH OF THESE IS ONE TREAT UNIT

choose 14 a week

- **I medium glass of wine**
- **300 ml (½ pint) beer, cider or lager**
- **double measure of spirits**
- **I Lo Bar or Halo bar**
- **I small bag of low-fat crisps or**
- **WeightWatchers Weavers**

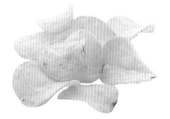

OR
EACH OF THESE IS TWO TREAT UNITS

choose 7 a week

- **I standard Wispa**
- **I Aero Milk Chunky**
- **medium slice of fruit cake**
- **one-third of an average 175 g (6 oz) garlic baguette**
- **any individual chilled dessert labelled '200 calories or less'.**

AT LUNCH AND EVENING MEAL YOU

- Reduce portion sizes of the high-fat, high-calorie foods and all red meat on your plate by between one-third and a half. See opposite for a comprehensive list of these foods.
- Continue to eat average portions of the carbohydrate foods on your plate (again see opposite for a list of these).
- Continue to eat average portions of any low- or medium-fat protein foods on your plate, excluding red meat which counts as high-fat (see below).
- Eat larger-than-average portions of vegetables and salad, as in your Unlimited list on the previous page.

You will reduce your calorie intake enough by doing this to lose between one and two pounds of weight a week. If you follow the guidelines, you will still have a full plate, you will still feel full and satisfied, and you will be getting a healthier diet while fitting in with the other members of the household, if necessary.

HIGH-CARBOHYDRATE FOODS
Continue to eat average portions

- Bread (all kinds), potatoes (plainly cooked), rice and other grains, pasta, white or wholewheat, sweet potatoes.

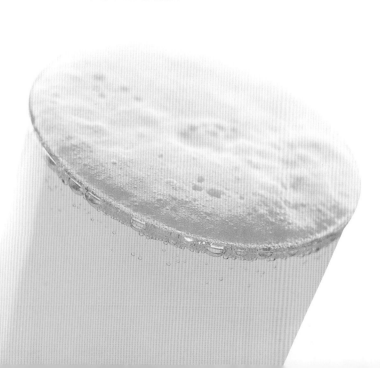

LOW- OR MODERATE-FAT, MODERATE-CALORIE PROTEIN FOODS
Continue to eat average portions

- Poultry (skin removed), fish, shellfish, eggs (plainly cooked), pheasant, venison, wild duck, guinea fowl, ostrich, lentils, pulses (including baked beans in tomato sauce), lentil soup.

HIGH-CALORIE, HIGH-FAT
Reduce portions by one-half to one-third

● Butter, margarine, suet, lard, pastry, blended vegetable oils, mayonnaise, pesto, coconut cream/milk.

● Cheddar and other hard cheeses, Stilton and other blue cheeses, all cream cheeses.

● Brie, Camembert.

● Pork pies, sausage rolls, quiches and other savoury pastries.

● Bacon, sausages, gammon, pork, crackling, lamb, beef, duck (except wild).

● Nuts, chips, deep-fried foods, taramasalata, peanut butter, meat pâtés.

VEGETABLES AND SALADS
Increase portion sizes

● All vegetables, except potatoes and sweet potatoes, plainly cooked.
● All salad items, except those in mayonnaise (treat as high-fat).
● Vegetables soups without added cream.

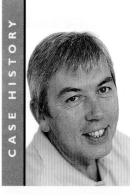

Noel leads an exceptionally busy working life on the road – he travels 30,000 miles a year and so wanted an eating programme that he could manage in these difficult circumstances. He also wanted ordinary family-type meals because when not on the road he is at home with his wife Lynne and they always eat together then. 'I've chosen the Portion Power Programme because it means I don't have to select special foods, but rather alter the balance of what I eat and cut down on portion sizes. My main weakness is for sweets, chocolate and junk foods, such as sausage rolls, so I shall have to make a list of alternative snacks that I can keep in the car!'

In the event, Noel managed to lose an amazing four inches off his middle in the 10 weeks. 'I cut right back on the high-calorie things on my plate and ate more vegetables. I snacked on fruit, which I quite like anyway, and treated myself to one Mars bar about three times a week, which seemed to keep my sweet tooth satisfied.'

FAT CONTROL

IF YOU ARE OVERWEIGHT, YOU HAVE BEEN SUPPLYING YOUR BODY WITH TOO MANY CALORIES FOR YOUR NEEDS. MANY PEOPLE FIND THAT THE MOST SUCCESSFUL WAY TO CUT THEIR CALORIE CONSUMPTION IS TO REDUCE THE OVERALL FAT CONTENT OF THEIR DIET BY AVOIDING ALL HIGH-FAT FOODS.

The main reason for this, as we discussed earlier, is that fat is much higher in calories than the other major nutrients, carbohydrate and protein. So cutting fat will save over twice the calories, while still allowing you to eat plenty.

The healthiest type of low-fat diet is one which cuts mainly saturated fats (found mostly in dairy and animal produce) and trans fats (found in commercial products, like margarine, cakes and biscuits) while still allowing you some polyunsaturated and mono-unsaturated fats in the diet. For more detail on the benefits of these, and more information on fats and good nutrition, see page 26.

On the Fat Control programme you will be eating plenty of carbohydrates (particularly complex carbohydrates), adequate amounts of low-fat protein, and it is important to eat a minimum of at least 5 portions of fruit and vegetables/salad a day. All fruit and non-starchy vegetables are unlimited on this diet.

As well as cutting fat, you will also be cutting sugar (without even trying, in most cases, as many of the high-fat foods are also high in sugar) and alcohol. That is because both of these are virtually 'empty' calories, and too much of either will hinder a weight-loss programme.

If you want to follow the Fat Control programme and don't need to lose weight, increase portion sizes and have extra snacks during the day of bananas, dried fruit and bread.

INSTRUCTIONS

• Every day you pick a Breakfast, a Light Meal and a Main Meal, plus two Mini Snacks to be eaten whenever you like.

• You also have a daily milk allowance, a list of Unlimited items and a weekly alcohol or chocolate allowance which is optional.

• Vary your choices as much as possible. If you have to eat out, turn to pages 50–51 for tips.

UNLIMITEDS

Eats:
• ALL vegetables, except potatoes or sweet potatoes, plainly cooked without added fat, unless a fat or oil allowance is mentioned within the meals.
• All fresh salad items.
• All fresh fruits, raw or baked or stewed, with a little fructose or artificial sweetener.
Note: It is vital to eat as many vegetables, fruits and salads as you can on a regular basis. Vary your choices but as bananas are the only starchy fruit limit them to 1–2 a day.

Drinks:
• Water, mineral water (try to get at least 4 large glasses of water a day as most other drinks don't hydrate you properly).
• Weak tea or coffee (with milk from allowance).
• Green tea, herbal teas.
• Hypotonic rehydrating 'sports drinks' containing no more than 4% sugars (check label).
• Calorie-free squashes and mixers.
Note: fruit juice contains a lot of calories and so is best used only once a day, diluted with water. Citrus juices are the best for vitamin C content.

Condiments:
Fresh or dried herbs and spices of all kinds, tomato purée and passata, Worcestershire sauce, light soy sauce, vinegars, low-fat stock cubes, ready-made stock.

MILK ALLOWANCE

• 200 ml (7 fl oz) skimmed or semi-skimmed milk for use in drinks or as a drink on its own.
• Any milk mentioned within the meals is extra to this.

ALCOHOL/CHOCOLATE ALLOWANCE

Every week you are allowed 7 units of alcohol
i.e. 7 medium glasses of table wine or half-pints of beer, lager or cider, or 7 measures of spirits *or* you can have 2 average chocolate bars instead.

MINI SNACKS

Every day have 2 mini snacks from the following – *also an ideal time to have some fruit*:

- **1 Quaker Harvest Apple and Raisin Chewy Bar.**
- **1 Shape Twinpot yoghurt or Mullerlight yoghurt.**
- **1 Boots Forest Fruits bar.**
- **2 dark rye Ryvitas with a little low-fat spread and Marmite.**
- **2 rice cakes each spread with a little runny honey.**
- **1 small handful of sunflower seeds or pine nuts.**
- **2–3 cold cooked new potatoes sprinkled with a little sea salt.**
- **1 Shape fromage frais with 3 pieces of dried ready-to-eat apricot.**
- **1 medium slice of malt loaf.**
- **1 mini pitta with 1 tablespoon tzatziki or hot tomato chilli dip.**

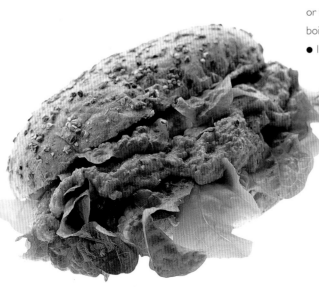

BREAKFASTS

Choose one a day of the following and add fruit to every breakfast if possible:

- 30 g (1 medium bowlful) any unsweetened breakfast cereal of choice, but whole-grain preferable (e.g. Weetabix, Shredded Wheat, All Bran) plus skimmed milk to cover; 1 medium slice of bread (preferably wholemeal or rye); a little low-fat spread if liked; low-sugar jam or marmalade or Marmite.
- 1 medium bowlful of porridge made with half water, half skimmed milk; 1 teaspoon brown sugar or a little honey; skimmed milk to cover if liked; 1 small slice of bread as before.
- 50 g (2 oz) no-added-sugar muesli, with skimmed milk to cover (please weigh the muesli).
- 1 medium bowlful of low-fat bio yoghurt with 25 g (1 oz) muesli sprinkled on it and a little runny honey. Do add chopped fruit or berries to this breakfast.
- 1 Shape Twinpot yoghurt, 1 large banana.
- 2 medium slices of rye bread with a little low-fat spread, low-sugar jam or marmalade, 1 Shape fromage frais.
- 1 medium slice of wholemeal or rye bread or toast; a little low-fat spread; 1 medium egg, boiled or poached.
- 1 Muller Crunch Corner yoghurt with one or two fruits.
- 200 g (7 oz) baked beans in tomato sauce on 1 medium slice of wholemeal toast, with a very little low-fat spread if liked.

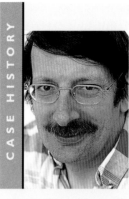

Chris Hall opted for the Fat Control Programme as he felt it was the plan that would most happily fit into his working and family life. 'On the Fat Control plan I can have most of the things that I enjoy – which are ethnic meals, fish and whole-grains and vegetables.' Chris's main areas to watch, we decided, were going to be his liking for sweet snacks, his alcohol intake and full-fat dairy produce.

After a few weeks Chris was finding it quite easy to stick to the programme, as he could see the weight coming off. 'It's great,' he said. 'I have cereal and semi-skimmed milk for breakfast, but have cut out toast and spread. For lunch I have a low-fat sandwich, such as chicken or a lower-fat cheese, plus salad on brown bread, or if entertaining I have fish or a rice dish instead of fatty meat. In the evening I enjoy pasta or a stir-fry with lots of vegetables and I have found I can still have a couple of glasses of wine. I've had to cut out my flapjacks and other sweet between-meal snacks, but I can't honestly say I've been hungry at all. All I really miss is steak and kidney pie!'

CHILLI TOMATO SAUCE

MAKES 2 PORTIONS *will freeze*
85 CALORIES AND 5 G FAT PER PORTION

1 dessertspoon olive oil

1 small-to-medium onion, finely chopped

1 garlic clove, crushed, or 1 level
teaspoon garlic purée

1 fresh green chilli, deseeded and finely
chopped *

400 g (14 oz) chopped Italian plum
tomatoes

1 dessertspoon tomato purée

1 teaspoon sun-dried tomato paste

dash of lemon juice

pinch of brown sugar

salt and black pepper

Heat the oil in a non-stick frying pan, add
the onion and stir-fry for a minute or two,
until translucent and tinged pale golden.
Add the garlic and chilli, and stir for
another minute.

Add the rest of the ingredients, bring to
simmer, cover and cook over a low heat
for 30 minutes, stirring once or twice.
Check the seasoning.

Serve with pasta, baked potato, etc. For a
creamier smoother sauce, purée in a
blender.

* *Red chilli will be hotter. If you like things
really hot, add the seeds too. If you can't
get fresh chilli, add a level teaspoon or so
of dried.*

Note: *add some sliced mushrooms to
the sauce for the last 10 minutes
of cooking for some low-fat
protein; or, for a more
substantial sauce, add
diced Quorn.*

LUNCHES

*Choose one a day of the following and don't
forget to add plenty of salad, fruit etc.*

● Home-made sandwich using 2 medium slices
of bread *or* 1 large bap, preferably wholemeal or
rye, very lightly spread with low-fat spread, if
used *or* with Hellmann's Light Mayonnaise if
preferred, and filled with unlimited salad items,
plus one of the following: 1 medium egg, hard-
boiled, and 1 teaspoon light mayonnaise / 100 g
(3½ oz) canned tuna in brine, well drained/ as
many prawns as you like, plus 1 teaspoon light
mayonnaise / 50 g (2 oz) cooked chicken or
turkey (no skin) plus 1 teaspoon mango
chutney / 2 average slices of extra-lean ham,
plus French mustard / 50 g (2 oz) poached
salmon, plus 1 teaspoon light mayonnaise or
pesto / 60 g (2½ oz) canned dressed crab,
plus 1 teaspoon light mayonnaise / 30 g
(1¼ oz) Brie or half-fat Cheddar or Roulé
(please weigh the cheese), plus 2 teaspoons
sweet pickle or other relish;
PLUS, with any above choice, some fruit and,
if liked, 1 whole can of WeightWatchers
Tomato or Minestrone Soup.

● 1 whole carton of New Covent Garden
chilled Tomato or Tomato and Lentil or Tuscan
Bean or Carrot and Coriander soup, 1 medium slice of bread or a roll. Fruit or yoghurt.

● 1 ready-made bought sandwich on wholemeal bread, containing 300 calories or less
and 10 g fat or less (check label).
PLUS fruit and a carton of
low-calorie yoghurt and, if
liked, a WeightWatchers
Tomato or Minestrone soup.

● 1 Boots Shapers Triple
Sandwich Pack; fruit.

● Prêt à Manger prawn,
chicken or vegetarian

crêpe, plus fruit and yoghurt or
WeightWatchers soup as above.

● Any ready-made fresh chilled salad (e.g.
M&S, Boots) containing 300 calories and 10 g
fat or less, plus fruit, yoghurt/soup as above.

● Salad (*serves 1):* mix together 6 tablespoons of leftover cooked rice or couscous
with 1 handful of chopped cooked turkey or
chicken or lean ham, plus chopped raw salad
vegetables, 25 g (1oz) chopped ready-to-eat
dried apricots, a few pine nuts or sunflower
seeds, all tossed in Waistline oil-free French
dressing *or* natural yoghurt and lemon juice.

● Salad (*serves 1):* 40 g (1½ oz) Feta cheese
(please weigh), crumbled, with tomato,
cucumber, green pepper, red onion, all
chopped, 4 chopped stoned black olives, 1
tablespoon real French dressing, 1 mini pitta
or 1 medium slice of rustic bread.

● 200 g (7 oz) baked beans in tomato
sauce on 1 medium slice of toast, topped
with 1 tablespoon grated half-fat cheese.

● 1 medium baked potato, topped with
4 tablespoons ready-made tzatziki *or* baked
beans *or* Chilli Tomato Sauce (*left*).

● 1 M&S 95% Fat-Free Stonebake Vegetable
Pizza.

EVENING MEALS

*Choose one a day of the following. Don't forget
to add plenty of vegetables in addition to any
mentioned within the meals.*

Note: *if you are not having your alcohol or
chocolate allowance you can have a spoonful of
olive or corn or groundnut oil for stir-frying, roasting, drizzling, or whatever, or a small knob of
butter, or you can have 25 g (1 oz) – please
weigh – full-fat cheese with or after your meal.
Have fresh fruit for dessert.*

● Average chicken breast portion, skin
removed and basted with a little ready-made

marinade mix (e.g. Schwartz or Lea & Perrins), baked or grilled; medium portion of potato, rice, couscous or pasta.

Tip: reconstitute couscous in vegetable stock or saffron rice stock (from a cube).

● Large white fish portion, cooked without fat (i.e. grilled, baked, griddled, steamed, poached, microwaved); medium portion of potato.

● Medium portion of oily fish (salmon, trout, mackerel, sardines, fresh tuna), cooked as above; medium portion potato, rice or pasta.

● 75 g (2¾ oz), dry weight, pasta of choice or 100 g (3½ oz) fresh pasta, boiled according to pack instructions and served with a large portion of Chilli Tomato Sauce (*see recipe opposite*) or half a jar of ready-made Italian Tomato Sauce, with a few sliced mushrooms.

● Medium portion of roast chicken, skin removed; 2 medium chunks of roast potato; vegetables; thin gravy skimmed of fat; 1 slice of crispy roast back bacon or small chipolata.

● Stir-fry of large amount of a variety of thinly sliced vegetables, with 100 g (3½ oz)

sliced lean chicken, turkey, pork or beef, with light soy sauce, dash of vinegar, honey or plum sauce, medium portion of plain boiled rice or egg-thread noodles or rice noodles.

● Large selection of vegetables suitable for roasting, e.g. aubergine, courgette, red pepper, red onion, tomatoes, garlic, brushed with a little olive oil and seasoned, placed in baking tray and roasted for 45 minutes, turning once; served on bed of couscous or rice or pasta, plainly cooked, plus 1 level tablespoon grated Parmesan cheese or similar.

● Any individual supermarket chilled ready-meal containing 450 calories or less and 20 g fat or less per portion if complete meal, or 250 calories and 15 g fat or less per portion if potato, rice, pasta or bread needs to be added to make a complete meal. Add plenty of salad, fruit, etc. Limit ready-meals to once or twice a week.

● 1 portion of Spicy Supper (*see recipe on the right*) with medium portion of plain boiled rice or 1 chapati.

Spicy Supper

Serves 2
325 calories per portion

300 g (10½ oz) potatoes

salt and black pepper

1 tablespoon groundnut oil

1 medium onion, chopped

1 garlic clove, crushed *or* 1 teaspoon
  garlic purée

1 dessertspoon good-quality curry
  powder of choice

about 5 tablespoons vegetable or
  chicken stock

1 tablespoon tomato purée

100 g (3½ oz) Quorn chunks *or* prawns
  or canned and drained brown lentils

300 g (10½ oz) frozen leaf spinach,
  defrosted and drained

100 ml (3½ fl oz) half-fat Total Greek
  yoghurt (or similar)

Peel the potatoes and cut into bite-sized chunks. Boil in lightly salted water until tender, about 10 minutes, then drain.
While the potatoes are cooking, heat the oil in a non-stick frying pan and add the onion, stirring, over a medium heat until soft. Add the garlic and curry powder and stir for a minute.
Add the stock mixed with the tomato purée, the Quorn or prawns or lentils and the potato chunks, bring to simmer and cook, stirring once or twice, for 15–20 minutes and adding a little more stock if the curry looks too dry (though it shouldn't be swimming).
Add the spinach, seasoning as necessary and yoghurt, stir for a few minutes to heat through and serve.

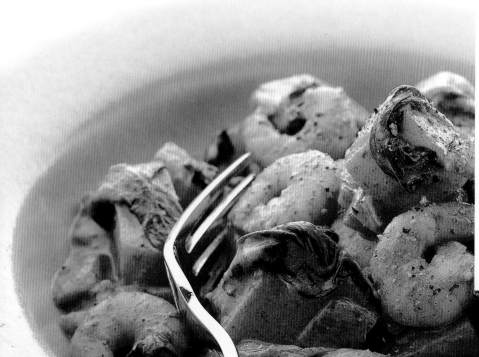

THE CARB-3 PROGRAMME

THIS IS THE IDEAL PROGRAMME FOR MEN WHO REALLY CAN'T DECIDE WHETHER THEY CAN LIVE WITHOUT LASHINGS OF CARBOHYDRATE FOODS, SUCH AS BREAD, POTATOES AND PASTA – OR WITHOUT THEIR REGULAR FIX OF PROTEIN, IN THE FORM OF THINGS LIKE MEAT OR CHEESE! WITH CARB-3 YOU CAN HAVE THE BEST OF BOTH WORLDS. THE ONLY CRITERION IS THAT YOU DON'T HAVE BOTH AT THE SAME TIME!

There is no mystery to how this programme works – you have three 'carb' days a week, on which you cut right back on protein, and four 'protein' days a week on which you cut right back on carbohydrates. You'll lose weight on the system because you're cutting calories overall, without having to weigh or measure anything. Once you get the hang of the programme, it is very simple. All you have to do is decide which are going to be your carb days, and stick to it. If you have to eat out, you will be able to find something suitable on most menus, whether it is a carb or protein day. And you'll be able to enjoy a wide range of foods.

If you would like to know more about carbohydrates, proteins and nutrition in general, turn to Nutrition in a Nutshell on pages 26–7.

INSTRUCTIONS
Applying to both Carb and Protein days

- Every day you will eat a Breakfast, a Light Lunch and an Evening Meal, plus two Mini Snacks a day.
- You also have a list of Unlimited items, a daily milk allowance, and a weekly alcohol allowance (optional).
- Just decide beforehand which days of the week you are going to go 'carb' and which 'protein', and choose your meals and Mini Snacks from the appropriate pages. All the carb choices appear on pages 41–3, all the protein choices on pages 44–5.
- It is best to alternate carb days with protein days if possible.

UNLIMITEDS
Same as in Fat Control programme, page 36, except bananas excluded on protein days.

MILK ALLOWANCE
Same as in Fat Control programme, page 36.

ALCOHOL ALLOWANCE
On Carb days only you are allowed up to 1 pint of beer, lager or cider, or 2 small glasses of wine or 1 double measure of spirits. No alcohol on protein days.

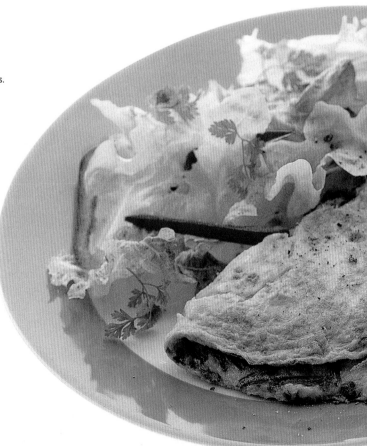

CARB DAYS

Have 3 a week. Don't forget
your unlimiteds (PLENTY of
vegetables, salad, fruit), milk
allowance, and alcohol
allowance if required.
Portion sizes are guides only –
eat enough to satisfy your
appetite and no more. Eat
slowly and chew thoroughly.
Bread, rice and pasta should
ideally be whole-grain.

BREAKFASTS

● 2 slices of bread or toast very lightly spread
with low-fat spread; low-sugar jam or marmalade or Marmite.

● I toasted tea-cake with low-fat spread and
jam or marmalade as above.

● Medium bowlful of Fruit 'n Fibre or
Shreddies or Branflakes or Oat Bran Flakes,
with enough skimmed milk to cover; I slice
of bread or toast with low-sugar jam or
marmalade.

● 2 Weetabix or Shredded Wheat with
skimmed milk to cover; I banana.

● Small-to-medium bowlful of no-added-sugar
muesli with skimmed milk or orange juice to
cover and plenty of fruit chopped in.

LIGHT LUNCHES

● Sandwiches – 2 or 3 slices of bread, lightly
spread with low-fat spread and filled with
either unlimited salad items plus a little
Hellmann's light mayonnaise, or with the
addition of Marmite OR Tartex vegetable,
yeast or mushroom pâté. You could also occasionally have your sandwich filled with honey
or pure fruit spread. Follow with a banana
(plus other fruit as liked).

● Grilled tomatoes on toast – 2 slices of toast
with a little low-fat spread, topped with unlimited grilled seasoned tomatoes. Fruit to follow.

● Stir-fried mushrooms on toast – stir-fry
plenty of mushrooms in a little olive or corn
oil and serve on 2 slices of toast. A little
Worcestershire or soy sauce adds flavour.
Fruit to follow.

● Take-away sandwich – Prêt à Manger vegetarian filled crêpe or salad sandwich from deli
(low-fat mayo), or roast veg baguette.

● Split pitta bread filled with chopped salad
items and French dressing. Large banana.

● Pasta salad: any deli pasta and vegetable (or
fruit) salad in French dressing. Some super-
markets and Boots also do ready
pasta salads.

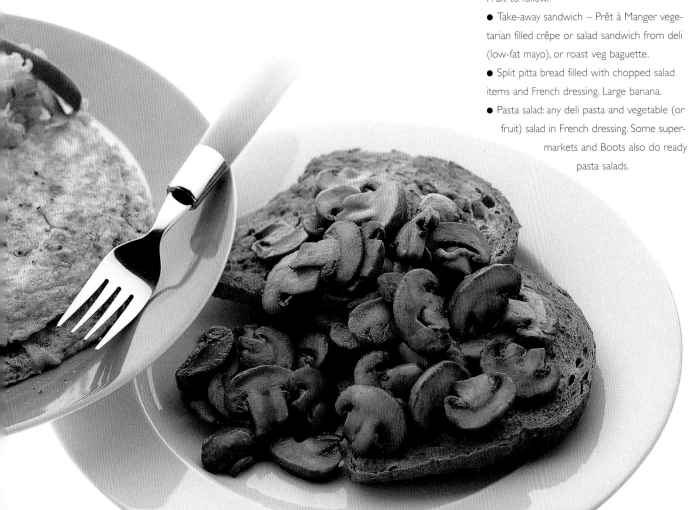

PEA AND POTATO SOUP

*Very healthy and so easy
and quick to make!*

SERVES 2 *will freeze*
175 CALORIES PER PORTION

250 g (9 oz) potatoes
500 ml (18 fl oz) vegetable stock
200 g (7 oz) peas (shelled weight)
    fresh or frozen
handful of freshly chopped flat-leaved
    parsley or mint
salt and black pepper
2 level tablespoons half-fat crème fraîche

Peel the potatoes, chop them and add to
the vegetable stock in a saucepan. Simmer
for 15 minutes, then add the peas and
herbs and simmer for a further 5 minutes.
Purée in a blender and season to taste.
Reheat and swirl in a level tablespoon of
half-fat crème fraîche per portion.

EVENING MEALS

● Baked potato with a knob of butter or
Greek yoghurt or a portion of Chilli Tomato
Sauce (see recipe on page 38); with large
salad and followed by fruit.

● Portion of Spicy Supper (see recipe on
page 39), excluding the Quorn, prawns or
lentils and adding 100 g (3½ oz) extra potato
instead; served with boiled rice or 1 chapati.

● Pasta of choice, boiled and topped with a
portion of Chilli Tomato Sauce (see recipe on
page 38) or ready-made Italian Tomato Sauce;
salad; fruit.

● Roast vegetables (see Fat Control evening
meals for details on page 39); rice, pasta or
baked potato.

● Bird's-Eye Vegetable Quarter Pounder with
potatoes, vegetables and relish.

● Linda McCartney Tikka Balti with Naan
(400-g size).

● 1 whole carton (600 ml / 1 pint) New
Covent Garden vegetable soup of choice
(e.g. Thai Spinach or Minestrone or Carrot
and Coriander or Plum Tomato), but not
including lentils or beans or cheese, *or* 1
portion home-made Pea and Potato Soup
(see recipe on the left). Serve with chunk of
bread or roll, and a banana to follow.

● 1 portion of spaghetti or tagliatelle with
Puttanesca Sauce (see recipe
opposite); banana.

● Selection of thinly
sliced vegetables
(as necessary)
stir-fried in a
little groundnut
oil, with soy sauce
and seasonings,
and served on a
bed of rice or
noodles.

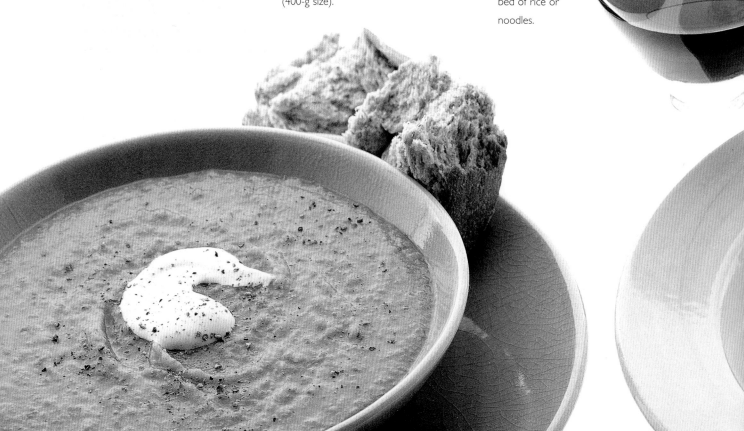

MINI SNACKS

Choose two a day:

- 1 banana
- 2 small digestive biscuits
- 1 crumpet with low-sugar jam
- 1 can of WeightWatcher's from Heinz vegetable soup.
- 1 Quaker Harvest Apple and Raisin Chewy Bar
- One 23-g pack of Butterkist popcorn
- 100 g (3½ oz) cold cooked new potatoes
- 1 mini pitta bread, sliced and dipped in Uncle Ben's Hot Salsa
- 1 medium slice of malt loaf

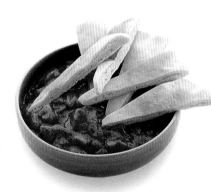

PUTTANESCA SAUCE

SERVES 2

160 CALORIES PER PORTION, EXCLUDING PASTA

2 dessertspoons olive oil
4 anchovy fillets in oil, drained and chopped
1 good garlic clove, crushed
200 g (7 oz) canned chopped tomatoes
5 stoned large black olives, chopped
1 dessertspoon drained capers
2 tablespoons finely chopped flat-leaved parsley
salt (if necessary) and black pepper
1 level tablespoon freshly grated Parmesan cheese

Heat the oil in a non-stick frying pan and add the anchovies and garlic. Stir for 30 seconds. Add the tomatoes and olives and simmer, covered, for 15 minutes. Then simmer, uncovered, for a further 10 minutes, stirring from time to time.
Add the capers and parsley for the last 5 minutes of cooking time. Add some black pepper. Check if the sauce needs salt – capers and olives are very salty, so it may not. Serve stirred well into pasta and topped with the Parmesan cheese.

Note: although Parmesan cheese is a high-protein food, you are using such a small amount in this dish that it won't upset your carb day.

PROTEIN DAYS

- Have 4 a week.
- Have a Breakfast, Light Lunch, Evening Meal and Two Mini Snacks a day.
- Don't forget your unlimited vegetables, salad, fruit (excluding banana on these days) and other Unlimiteds, as well as your milk allowance.
- Portion sizes are a guide only – eat enough to satisfy your appetite and no more.

BREAKFASTS

Choose one a day of the following:

- 1 large egg, boiled (hard-boiled if preferred); 1 dark rye Ryvita; fruit.
- 1 medium bowlful of low-fat natural bio yoghurt with up to 2 fruits, plus 1 teaspoon of runny honey. Small handful of chopped shelled walnuts or sunflower seeds.
- 1 Shape Twinpot yoghurt; fruit.
- 1 Mullerlight yoghurt; fruit.
- Grilled kipper fillets.
- 2 slices of extra-lean back bacon, grilled, with grilled tomatoes and baked beans.

LIGHT LUNCHES

Choose one a day of the following:

- Large mixed salad with oil-free French dressing, or a small amount of ordinary French dressing, or a dash of olive oil mixed with lemon juice. The salad can include avocado, nuts, seeds, extra-lean chopped ham or cooked chicken or prawns. You can also add chopped fruit or a couple of chopped dried apricots or peaches.
- 2 medium eggs, hard-boiled; 1 dark rye Ryvita; large mixed salad; fruit.
- 1 triangle of Camembert or 50 g (2 oz) Brie; large mixed salad; 1 dark rye Ryvita; fruit.
- Three-bean salad: mix together cooked green beans, red kidney beans and borlotti or flageolet or butter beans or cooked brown lentils or chickpeas – with unlimited crunchy salad items, chopped, plus chopped fresh tomato, all tossed in oil-free French dressing, served with green salad. Fruit to follow.
Note: You can use a can of mixed beans if you like.
- Tuna and prawn ready-made salad from Prêt à Manger; fruit.
- Can of tuna in brine, well drained; mixed salad with dressing; fruit.
- Prawn cocktail: bed of shredded lettuce topped with cooked peeled king prawns or mixed seafood, if preferred; plus slices of avocado, if liked, topped with light mayonnaise mixed half and half with low-fat bio yoghurt and lemon juice, with a dash of tomato purée mixed in and a dash of chilli sauce too; fruit.
- Crudités and dip: selection of batons of raw veg, e.g. carrot, spring onions, celery, peppers, mushrooms, with tzatziki (bought, or mix bio yoghurt with chopped cucumber, onion, garlic and mint) or with hummus or Mexican salsa, or with any Iceland 95% fat-free dip.

MINI SNACKS

Choose two a day of the following:

- Shape fruit yoghurt
- Mullerlight yoghurt
- Shape Twinpot
- 25 g (1 oz) Edam or Brie or Port Salut cheese on 1 dark rye Ryvita
- 1 medium egg, hard-boiled
- Small handful of shelled nuts (unsalted)
- Small handful of sunflower seeds or pine nuts
- 1 tablespoon hummus with 1 sliced raw carrot or celery stalk

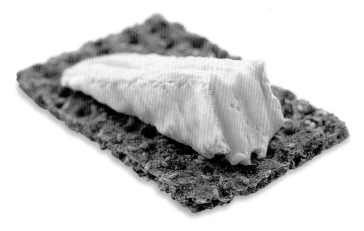

- M&S Layered Salad with Chicken or Prawns or Salmon; fruit.
- Lentil soup, bought or home-made; fruit.
- I whole carton of New Covent Garden Tuscan Bean or Broccoli with Stilton or Vegetable with Peanut or Smoked Haddock Chowder or Moroccan Chickpea and Spinach soup; fruit.

EVENING MEALS

Choose one a day of the following. Don't forget to add plenty of salad/vegetables:

- Lean beef steak, grilled or dry-fried, band of fat removed; selection of vegetables or large salad.
- Roast chicken or turkey; selection of vegetables (baked with olive oil if liked); thin gravy.

- Roast lean beef or leg of lamb or pork; selection of vegetables (baked with olive oil if liked); thin gravy.
- Chicken breast portion, skin removed, basted with a ready-made baste suitable for grilling (e.g. Baste and Go), grilled or baked or microwaved.
- Large white fish, cooked plainly or with a little fat; spoonful of tartare or hollandaise sauce, or light mayonnaise if liked.
- Medium portion of oily fish, cooked plainly or with a little fat.
- Omelette made from 2 large or 3 small eggs, a little water, small knob of butter, herbs or chopped lean ham to fill; large salad.
- I portion of Spiced Salmon with Lentils (see recipe on right).

Note: any evening meal can be served with stir-fried vegetables.

SPICED SALMON WITH LENTILS

SERVES 2
450 CALORIES PER PORTION

I tablespoon groundnut oil

I small onion, finely chopped

I garlic clove, crushed

I level tablespoon garam masala

200 g (7 oz) canned drained green lentils

300 g (10½ oz) canned chopped tomatoes

100 ml (3½ fl oz) fish stock (from cube or fresh chilled)

salt and black pepper

2 salmon fillets, each about 100 g (3½ oz)

I tablespoon half-fat crème fraîche

Heat the oil in a non-stick frying pan and sauté the onion for a few minutes until soft and just turning golden. Add the garlic and garam masala and stir for half a minute.
Add the lentils, tomatoes, stock and seasoning, stir again and simmer gently for 15 minutes, stirring once or twice.
When you have a rich sauce, add the salmon fillets and simmer until they are just cooked, about 5 minutes.
Put the salmon on serving plates and stir the crème fraîche into the sauce. Serve the sauce with the salmon.

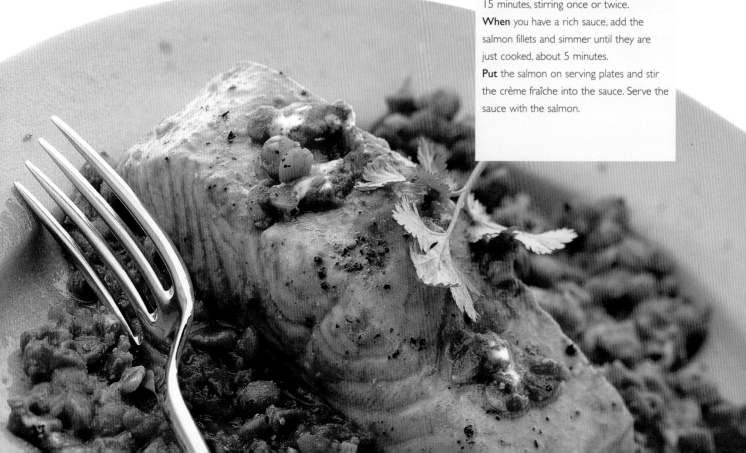

THE DETOX PROGRAMME

AS EXPLAINED OPPOSITE, THIS DETOX SYSTEM IS VERY GENTLE AND GRADUAL, AND DOESN'T REQUIRE YOU TO FAST. A GOOD DETOX PROGRAMME WILL HELP YOU FEEL AND LOOK BETTER IN SEVERAL WAYS EXPLAINED BELOW.

TEN TIPS FOR EFFICIENT DETOXING

❶ Eat as much of your fruit and vegetables raw as you can.

❷ Buy organic food if you can.

❸ Buy the best-quality food you can.

❹ If possible, know the source of your food.

❺ Make sure the food that you buy is as fresh as possible.

❻ Make sure that the food you buy is stored as well as possible – in cool, dark conditions, properly wrapped.

❼ Drink plenty, especially water and herbal teas.

❽ Take plenty of fresh herbs in your diet, especially the herbs mentioned in the programme.

❾ Eat 'little and often'.

❿ Follow your exercise programme (see Section 3) properly to aid elimination of toxins.

● You will be cutting down on – or out – foods and drinks high in any likely toxins – chemical food additives, hormones, residues, etc.

● You will be cutting down on, or out, highly refined foods.

● You will be increasing your intake of natural foods, drinks and herbs that help the liver (which processes toxins) and the lymph system (which removes the released toxins from the system) and with fluid elimination.

● You will be increasing your natural fibre intake, which will help speed up elimination.

● You will be cutting out most of the foods most commonly associated with allergies and food intolerance.

● You will be increasing your intake of antioxidant foods, drinks and herbs.

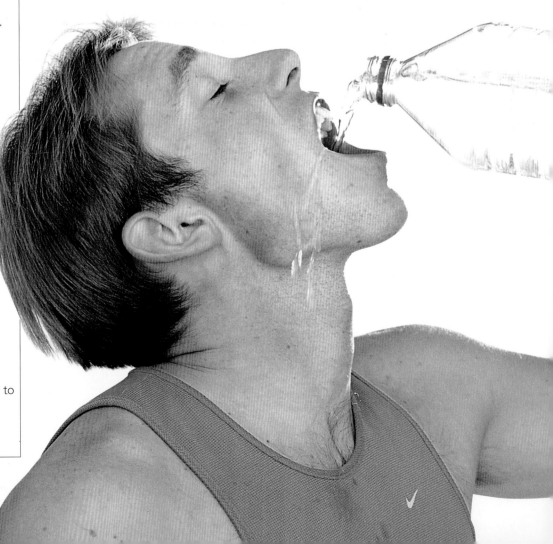

Antioxidants help mop up the extra 'free radicals' (which contribute to the ageing process and may increase risk of heart disease and cancers) that are produced during a detox regime. Some of these antioxidant foods also have powerful anti-viral, anti-fungal and anti-bacterial effects.

● You will lose weight easily, if necessary, as the Detox Programme is naturally lower in calories than the average normal Western-style diet, while being high in essential nutrients and fatty acids.

● After a few weeks on the Detox Programme you should find a notice-able improvement in the appearance of your skin, eyes and gums. You should also feel alert and energized.

Following the programme . . .

. . . is very easy. Every week you simply follow the instructions for that week, avoiding certain foods and taking more of others. The programme gradually goes deeper into 'detox' for the first 3 weeks, remains at that level for a further 5 weeks and then, for the last 2 weeks of the programme, gradually re-introduces foods. You will, however, need to spend plenty of time sorting out your storecupboard, fridge and freezer, and restocking on items for your detox. The diet requires a very high level of fresh and natural produce, especially vegetables, salad and fruit. You will also need to be in the right frame of mind to follow this plan, but if it was your preferred choice (see page 31) you should be fine. Also, see the tips box opposite for how to get the most out of your detox.

Unlimited

Unlimited throughout the detox is water and mineral water. You should aim to drink at least 2.25 litres (4 pints) a day.

WEEK I

Avoid:
● Alcohol.
● Smoking.
● Meat (excluding poultry and game).
● Full-fat cheeses, such as Cheddar, Stilton, cream cheese.
● Cream and full-cream milk.
● Added sugar in tea, on cereal, etc.
● Added salt, in cooking at table, etc.
● Any convenience food containing chemical additives (e.g. packet soups, sauces, dried mixes, ambient desserts). Read the labels.

Eat/drink more:
● Fresh fruit – aim for at least 2 portions a day.
● All vegetables, particularly leafy green vegetables such as Brussels sprouts and dark cabbage, broccoli, peas, green beans, broad beans and sweetcorn.
● Fish.
● Water.

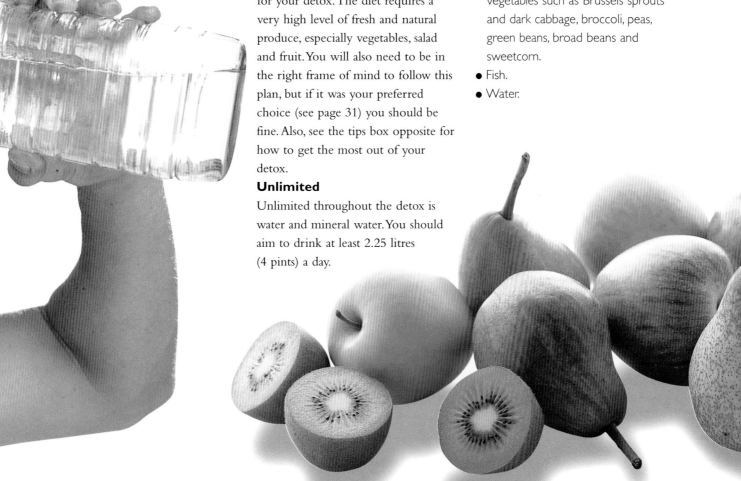

HERBS FOR DETOXING

Rosemary a stimulant, tonic and anti-bacterial.
Dandelion aids liver function and helps fluid elimination (acts as a diuretic).
Burdock aids liver function and acts as a natural laxative.
Nettle a natural diuretic.
Parsley a diuretic, helps digestive system.
Mint helps digestive system and liver function.
Oregano stimulates the lymph system and is anti-bacterial.
Thyme a stimulant, anti-bacterial.
Garlic antioxidant, anti-bacterial, anti-fungal, anti-viral.

WEEK 2

Avoid:

- Everything as Week 1.
- Refined cereal products, e.g. white bread, white pasta, white rice.
- All savoury snack foods, such as salted nuts, crisps.
- All chocolate and products containing chocolate, and all sweets.
- All hard fats, including butter, margarine, lard, suet and low-fat spreads.
- All caffeine-containing drinks, including coffee, tea, cola.
- Commercial desserts, cakes, gâteaux, biscuits, savoury crackers and pastries.
- Savoury pastry items, e.g. pies, pasties, tarts.

Eat/drink more:

- Everything as Week 1.
- Raw salads dressed with extra-virgin olive oil and lemon or lime juice.
- Citrus fruits; berry fruits; melon; pineapple; plums; cherries; red grapes; apples.
- Whole-grain cereals, particularly brown rice.
- Red, orange and yellow vegetables, e.g. sweet peppers, squashes, carrots, tomatoes.
- Onions and leeks.
- Garlic.

Note: if you are losing too much weight (or are losing weight quicker than 2 pounds a week) UP your intake of the dried fruits listed in Week 3, UP your intake of plant oils and starchy vegetables, such as potatoes and sweet potatoes, UP your intake of avocados, nuts, seeds and bananas.

WEEK 3

Avoid:

- Everything as Weeks 1 and 2.
- Eggs.
- All cheese.
- Poultry, game and all animal flesh.
- All long-life products and canned fruits and vegetables, except tomatoes and pulses in water.
- Commercial squashes, fizzy drinks, mixers.

Eat/drink more:

- Everything as Weeks 1 and 2.
- Oily fish – preferably organic, salmon, herring, mackerel, trout, tuna, sardines.
- Pulses – lentils (brown or green), chickpeas, butter beans, flageolets, etc. and beansprouts.
- Fresh herbs – especially thyme, rosemary, oregano, basil, sage.
- Dried figs, prunes, apricots, preferably organic (*not* containing sulphur).

WEEKS 4–8

Avoid:

- Everything as Weeks 1–3.
- All wheat-based products, including wheat bread, pasta, crispbreads and wheat-containing breakfast cereals.
- All dairy produce, including milk of all kinds, yoghurt of all kinds.

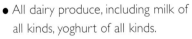

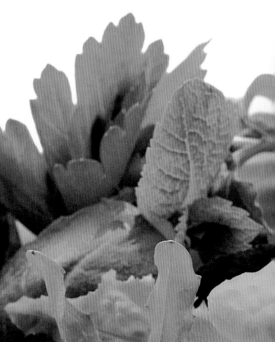

WAYS TO TAKE HERBS

● As a hot herbal tea – chop herb leaves as necessary and pour boiling water over, using about 2 level teaspoons of fresh herb per person. Leave for a few minutes to steep, strain and serve.

● As a decoction (used for roots and woody stems, such as dandelion or burdock root): chop the root and simmer in a saucepan with water to cover for 30 minutes or so, until the liquid is reduced by one-third. Strain and drink (or you could even use a stock for soup).

● Chopped, fresh, into salads – good for this are basil, parsley, sorrel, lovage, coriander and garlic.

● Stirred into vegetables soups and casseroles – good for this are coriander, parsley, oregano, thyme, garlic.

● All shellfish and any non-organic (or non-wild) fresh fish.
● Strawberries.

Eat/drink more of:
● Organic dark rye bread.
● Organic calcium-fortified soya milk and soya yoghurt.
● Organic porridge and oat-based muesli.
● Green tea, herbal teas (preferably home-made, *see box left*).
● Pure plant oils, especially olive oil, groundnut oil, corn oil, all preferably used raw in salads and garnishes.
● Keep eating plenty of fresh fruit and vegetables at every meal, especially leafy-green and dark-green vegetables and red, orange and yellow vegetables. Mostly raw or lightly cooked, but also use in soups and stir-fries.
● Garlic.
● Potatoes and all other root vegetables (organic).
● Avocados.
● All fresh nuts, especially walnuts and Brazils.
● Seeds – e.g. sunflower seeds, sesame seeds, pine nuts and pumpkin seeds.

WEEKS 9 AND 10
Reintroduce into your diet:
● Eggs.
● Low-fat dairy produce (skimmed milk, yoghurt, low-fat cheeses).
● Organic poultry and game.
● Whole-grain wheat bread and other whole-grain wheat products (if no allergic/intolerant response).
● Strawberries (if no allergic/intolerant response).
● Shellfish (if no allergic/intolerant response) in moderation.

Note: If you can't find a particular food mentioned, either singly or as part of a food group, whether as something to be avoided or as something to eat more of, assume you can include it in your diet in moderate amounts during the programme. Use your common sense!

IN FUTURE

Continue to try to eat the bulk of your menus as you have learnt over the past weeks. Add a little organic animal flesh, if you like, plus the occasional glass of good-quality alcohol – a little of what you fancy, etc. – but try to avoid, most of the time, the high-additive, high-salt, high-sugar, high-hard-fat diet you used to eat.

Once every few months or so you can repeat the 'hard core' of the Detox diet – Weeks 3 and 4 – to refresh your palate and mini detox your body.

EATING OUT WITHOUT GUILT

I DEFY ANYONE TO FOLLOW A 10-WEEK PROGRAMME WITHOUT EATING OUT AT LEAST A FEW TIMES IN THE PROCESS. HERE'S HOW TO FIT BUSINESS AND SOCIAL EATING INTO YOUR DIET PROGRAMME WITHOUT HAVING TO SUFFER GUILT PANGS – OR A NON-SHRINKING WAISTLINE.

**PICK
A RESTAURANT
TO MATCH
YOUR EATING
PROGRAMME**

If you're on the
**PORTION POWER
PROGRAMME**
Go for: New British;
New French;
Japanese.

If you're on the
LOW-FAT PROGRAMME
Go for: Japanese;
fish restaurant;
Californian; Pacific Rim cuisine;
good-quality Chinese;
New British.

If you're on the
CARB-3 PROGRAMME

On Carb days
choose
Indian, Italian, vegetarian.

On Protein days
choose
carvery, tandoori house,
fish restaurant.

If you're on the
DETOX PROGRAMME
Go for: whole-food restaurants;
vegetarian restaurants;
fish restaurants.

If your work, coupled with an active social life, requires you to eat out on a regular basis – perhaps almost every day – then, unless you know the best places to go, the best things to choose and what to avoid, you will undoubtedly find the results on your waistline. The tips here will help you to do that.

● Where to go? If the choice is yours, pick a restaurant where they know you and you know the menu. Avoid like the plague restaurants which serve only minuscule portions of vegetables. It is, however, quite a good idea to patronize places – of which there are many – that serve minuscule portions of everything else. The kind of restaurant my husband always complains is bad value for money may be just perfect for you, especially if you're following the Portion Power plan! If you are a regular, many places will serve you things your way – say, without added butter garnish, without rich sauces. Unless the restaurant is classic French variety or a greasy spoon, many of the dishes on the menu will be fairly low in calories and fat anyway – it's just a matter of picking the right ones. The box opposite will help you spot the better bets both for calories and fat. If in doubt, ask for more details about the dish's ingredients and how it is prepared.
● How many courses? If it is a business lunch, there is usually no obligation on

you to wade through three courses. Most people will agree that a light starter and a light main course will sustain you but not leave you feeling sluggish all afternoon.

When eating out in the evening, either for business or pleasure, it seems more usual to go for the whole works, but even then you can choose wisely and cut calories in other ways too.
● How? Well, skip the pre-meal nibbles. Avoid nuts and crisps – mega-calories, fat and salt. Skip anything other than a small roll before your meal arrives and forget all about the butter dish, garlic bread – anything smothered in fat. Choose at least one course consisting mainly of fruit or salad – preferably two, e.g. a light salad starter and a fruit salad or fresh fruit for dessert. Avoid second helpings of all courses (expect plain cooked veg) and

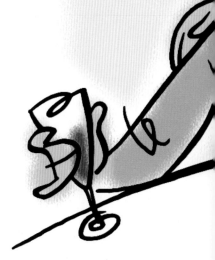

cut back on the amount of alcohol you consume.

● How? Drink plenty of water at the start of your evening – much alcohol, especially wine and beer, is consumed because you are thirsty. Sip don't gulp, and put your glass down between sips.

Have water in a large glass by your alcohol glass and have alternate sips from that. If it's lunch time, few people will mind if you don't drink alcohol at all. Claim a heavy afternoon's workload as an opt-out.

● If you're not hungry after your main course but fancy the sound of one of the desserts, try to persuade someone else to have it and have just one or two mouthfuls of theirs – most desserts really are stacked full of fat and calories, even innocent-looking small puds like crème brûlée and those tiny chocolate pots. Pastries, cheesecakes, lemon tarts – are all fairly much once-in-a-blue-moon treats too.

● If it's your birthday or anniversary – eat what you like and enjoy it without feeling guilty. Everyone needs a blow-out now and then!

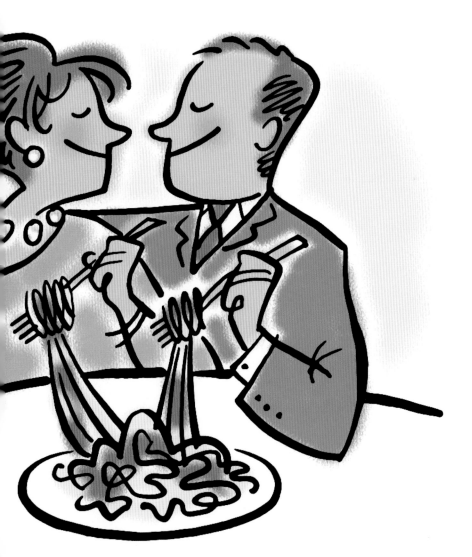

GOOD BETS FOR STARTERS:

MELON, plain or with Parma ham
MUSHROOMS À LA GRECQUE
(in tomato sauce not garlic butter)
CLEAR SOUP – e.g. many Chinese soups
or consomme
ASPARAGUS with a drizzle of olive oil
ARTICHOKE SALAD (minimal dressing)
CRUDITÉS and TZATZIKI.
Avoid most of the time:
meat-based pâtés, things in garlic butter;
savoury tarts, anything in mayonnaise;
anything with cheese;
any starter with meat in it; pasta.

GOOD BETS FOR MAIN COURSES:

GRILLED FISH; ROAST GAME
OR POULTRY
GRILLED OR BAKED LEAN LAMB CUTLETS
SMALL PLAIN COOKED LEAN STEAK
PASTA with tomato sauce; pasta with clams;
PASTA PRIMAVERA
TANDOORI-BAKED CHICKEN, VEGETABLE BALTI,
PLAIN RICE, CHAPATI
STIR-FRIES based on vegetables and
tofu or prawns
GRILLED VEGETABLES AND COUSCOUS
CHILLI PRAWNS.
Avoid most of the time:
rich cream and cheese-based sauces; pastry;
fatty cuts of meat; anything deep-fried;
coconut cream-rich curries; pizza with hefty
cheese/meat topping.

GOOD BETS FOR AFTERS:

FRESH FRUIT
FRUIT SALAD
FRUIT-FILLED FILO CASES
SORBET
PEARS IN RED WINE
BAKED PEACHES.
Avoid most of the time:
rich cream and chocolate confections; pies,
pastries, gâteaux and profiteroles;
cheese and biscuits.

getting physical

People who exercise maintain a youthful appearance for much longer.

exercise keeps you young

This section is all about how to get, or keep, your body fit and in good shape. How to make sure that your muscles, your bones, your joints, your ligaments and your cardiovascular system are all in as good working order as possible from now onwards. The reason this is important (for anyone, but especially those over the age of 40) is that, without a fit body, you will look (and feel) old before your time.

Let's start with looks. People who exercise really do maintain a youthful appearance for much longer, for several reasons. Regular activity helps to burn up calories, thus helping to keep middle-aged paunch and weight gain at bay. Exercise of all kinds also helps to keep your body shapely and firm. Once past your 20s, if you don't exercise, your muscle mass – and therefore strength and tone – will start to decline. With regular exercise, however, it is possible to maintain peak muscle mass well into old age – with a flat stomach, strong shoulders, the lot.

Perhaps the biggest giveaway of age is how you walk. To my mind, old age's image is of a shuffling, bent-over, stiff figure with all vitality gone. A sad picture that can mostly be avoided, not only by strength and stamina work – but by regular stretching and suppling exercise. Most men forget all about this aspect of exercise but it, too, is vital to avoid atrophied muscles and inflexible joints and ligaments.

Exercise also oxygenates your whole body, improving circulation and therefore the appearance of your skin. It may even help prevent baldness by increasing blood flow to the scalp.

Now on to how you feel. From digestive disorders to heart disease, the list of problems that can be overcome or minimized with exercise is almost endless, as you will discover overleaf. Activity can even improve your brainpower!

In other words, exercise keeps you young. If you do nothing else – begin to get moving NOW. It's never too late to start.

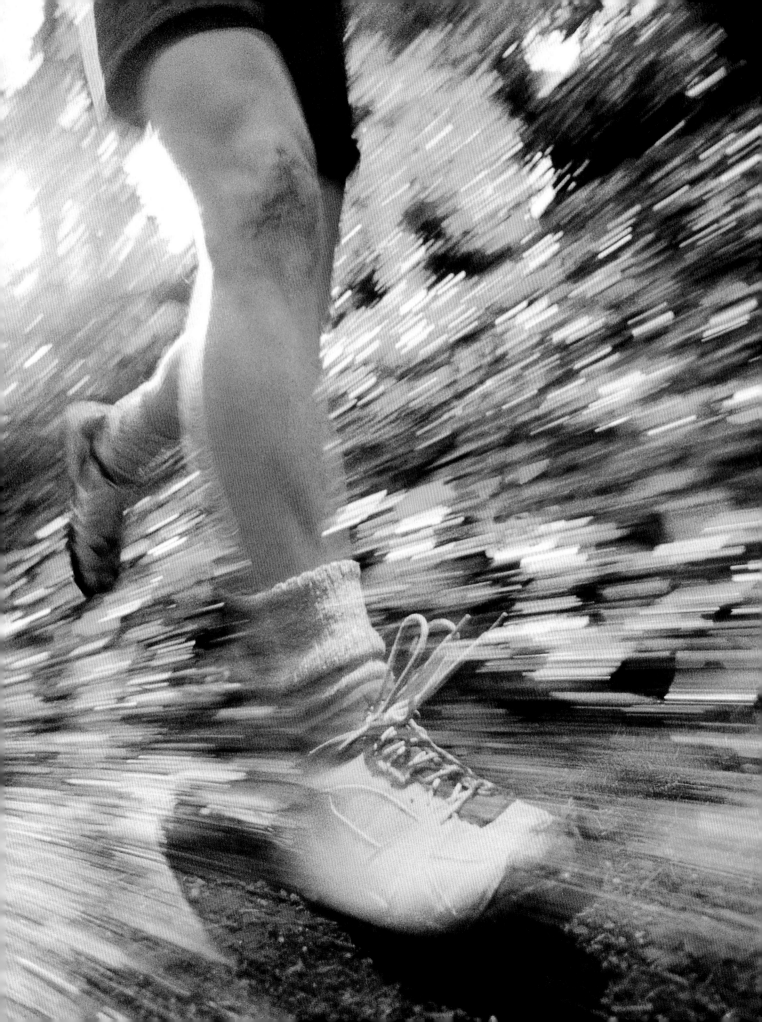

THE HOME CIRCUITS

EVEN IF YOU HAVEN'T EXERCISED FOR YEARS, IT IS NEVER TOO LATE TO START.

THE HOME CIRCUITS ARE THE IDEAL PLACE TO BEGIN.

GENERAL INSTRUCTIONS FOR THE HOME CIRCUITS

1 Check with your doctor if you have any doubt about your ability to begin one of the Home Circuits or if you have a medical condition.

2 Start on the correct Home Circuit for you.

3 Make sure you have everything you may need for your circuit.

4 Read through the exercises and make sure you understand them.

5 Read the At-a-Glance Circuit Chart and, if necessary, copy it out on a large sheet of card, to make sure you do the programme in the correct order and do the right number of sets (repeats of each exercise).

6 Wear suitable comfortable clothing – e.g. T-shirt and shorts or tracksuit bottoms, and comfortable supportive trainers and socks.

7 Don't skip the warm-up, the warm-up stretches or the cool-down. It is when you don't warm up and cool down properly that you may suffer aches the next day, or even injury, especially if you haven't exercised in a long time.

8 Sets given are average. If you are very unfit you may, at least for some of the exercises, have to stop before you have completed all the reps (repeats) for the required number of sets. You should work the muscle that is in training to the point where it is tired and beginning to tremble slightly, but you should not go beyond that point. Your strength and stamina will soon improve, so that you will soon be doing the amount stated.

9 The length of the Skip or Step sessions given are average. If you are very unfit you may find that, at first, you can't do the time stated, especially with skipping, which is very tough. You will soon build up to the time stated if you exercise regularly.

10 Breathe normally throughout unless otherwise stated.

11 Don't exercise after a heavy meal or when ill.

HOW FIT DO YOU WANT TO BE?

In 10 weeks a great deal can be achieved, and you don't need to feel you have to get super-fit – running marathons and the like – to achieve benefits in the areas mentioned above. Moderate increases in fitness levels produce excellent results.

HOW DO YOU BEGIN?

Having found out your Real Age (using the Assessments on pages 10–17) and having read the general instructions below, you can begin on your correct fitness programme – either Home Circuit 60+ (page 56), Home Circuit 50+ (page 60) or Home Circuit 40+ (page 64) – and see benefits almost straight away. The At-a-Glance Circuit Chart opposite shows you what each circuit consists of, how long you should spend on each element of it, and in what order they should be tackled. As the weeks progress, from time to time you will reassess your Real Age, as instructed in the schedules at the back of the book, and as your Real Age lowers you can also progress to the harder Home Circuits.

In addition to your Home Circuit, which should be done three times a week (as detailed in the schedules), you will also be doing regular Outdoor Exercise as described on pages 70–1 in this section. If you want to add on any other form of activity, read the section on Sport for All (pages 72–3), and if you have any queries on exercise in general you will find answers to the questions we are most often asked on pages 74–5.

This section of the book has been compiled with the help of top personal trainer Rob Lander, who models the exercises for Home Circuit 40+. His colleague Eddie Butler models the exercises for Home Circuits 50+ and 60+.

The At-a-Glance Circuit Charts

This shows you the order in which to do the exercises, plus the repeats/time to aim for.

EXERCISE	60+	50+	40+
Warm-up	2 mins	2 mins	2 mins
Warm-up Stretches	1 min	1 min	1 min
Skip or Step	1 min	2 mins	4 mins
Lateral Raises	1 set /16 reps	2 sets /32 reps	3 sets /48 reps
Bicep Curls	1 set /16 reps	2 sets /32 reps	3 sets /48 reps
Skip or Step	1 min	2 mins	4 mins
Squats	1 set /16 reps	2 sets /32 reps	3 sets /48 reps
Triceps Dips	1 set /16 reps	2 sets /32 reps	3 sets /48 reps
Skip or Step	1 min	2 mins	4 mins
Abs 1	1 set /16 reps	2 sets /32 reps	3 sets /48 reps
Abs 2	1 set /16 reps	2 sets /32 reps	3 sets /48 reps
Press-ups	1 set /16 reps	2 sets /32 reps	3 sets /48 reps
Gluteals *	1 set /16 reps	2 sets /32 reps	3 sets /48 reps
Cool-down Stretches	3–4 mins	3–4 mins	3–4 mins
Total time taken * *	**20 mins**	**25 mins**	**30 mins**

* For the 40+ Programme, Gluteal Curls are replaced with Lunges, which you can do after the Squats, if you prefer.

* * This is a rough guide only -- you may need longer than this.

FIVE GOOD REASONS TO EXERCISE

For your heart: stamina-building exercise, such as walking, cycling, jogging, which increases the fitness of your heart and lungs, will not only help to prevent cardiovascular disease, the biggest male killer, but also help stave off tiredness and feeling sluggish and 'foggy'.

For your bones and joints: weight-bearing exercise (e.g. walking for legs, free weights work for arms) helps to maintain bone density and prevent osteoporosis. Keeping active and supple helps to minimize arthritis and general 'aches and pains' that can often accompany getting older.

For a good night's sleep: research shows that people who exercise regularly suffer from less insomnia than people who don't. The best type of exercise to improve the quality of sleep is aerobic (stamina-building) exercise, such as walking.

For mental health: regular exercise decreases negative stress and is a powerful aid to relaxation, releasing hormones to help calm you down and alleviate depression. It also increases alertness and memory and has been shown to help prolong the onset of Alzheimer's disease.

For your digestive system: exercise improves the efficiency of the digestive system, speeding the passage of food through the gut and helping to eliminate constipation. It also decreases fluid retention and increases the flow of lymph to help the body rid itself of toxins (such as alcohol and nicotine).

HOME CIRCUIT 60 +

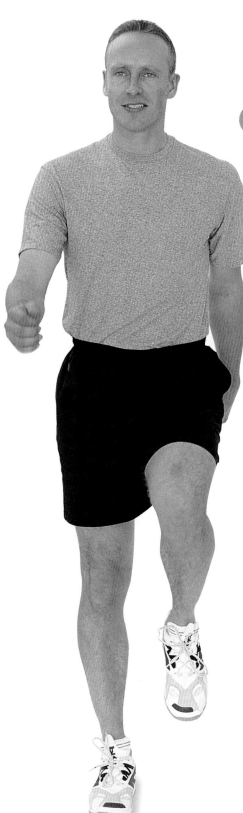

1 Warm-up:
March on the spot for 2 minutes, gradually raising your knees higher and higher and pumping your arms harder. Don't stop until you feel pleasantly warm and can feel your heart-rate beginning to rise.

2 Warm-up Stretches:
Do the Quad Stretch, Hamstring Stretch and Calf Stretch as described on page 68, holding each stretch for a slow count of 10.

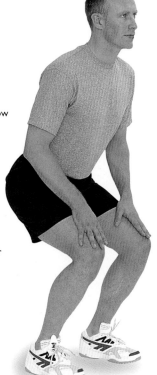

3 Skip or Step for 1 minute
Skip: skip lightly on the spot at a moderate pace, breathing steadily. This will raise your heart-rate. Check posture is good – stomach in, back erect.
Step: step up and down on a 25-cm (10-inch) step or stair or heavy-weight box (UP right, UP left, DOWN right, DOWN left; then UP left, UP right, DOWN left, DOWN right), landing on the floor a few inches from the edge of the step each time. Breathe steadily, feel heart-rate rise. Check posture – stomach in, leaning slightly forward.

7 Squats _For thighs and gluteals_
Stand with feet hip-width apart and toes pointing forwards, hands lightly resting on thighs, in a good posture position. Now slowly bend the knees without tipping forward, feeling your weight through the heels as if sitting back on a chair, and feeling your gluteal (buttock) muscles and thighs working. Hold for a second as far down as you can go (to a maximum of 90°), then slowly return to the starting position. Repeat 16 times for one set.

❶ CHECK: IS THIS THE RIGHT PROGRAMME FOR YOUR REAL AGE (SEE PAGES 16–17)?

❷ HAVE YOU READ THE GENERAL INSTRUCTIONS ON PAGE 54 AND THE AT-A-GLANCE CIRCUIT CHART ON PAGE 55?

❸ FOLLOW THE NUMBERS AROUND THESE FOUR PAGES FOR DETAILED INSTRUCTIONS ON THE EXERCISES THAT FORM YOUR HOME CIRCUIT.

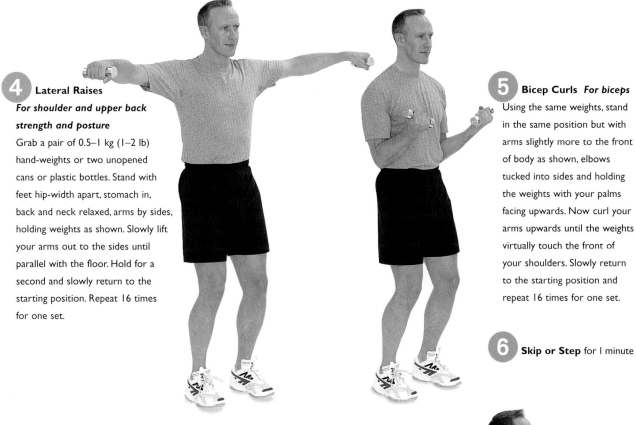

④ Lateral Raises

For shoulder and upper back strength and posture

Grab a pair of 0.5–1 kg (1–2 lb) hand-weights or two unopened cans or plastic bottles. Stand with feet hip-width apart, stomach in, back and neck relaxed, arms by sides, holding weights as shown. Slowly lift your arms out to the sides until parallel with the floor. Hold for a second and slowly return to the starting position. Repeat 16 times for one set.

⑤ Bicep Curls *For biceps*

Using the same weights, stand in the same position but with arms slightly more to the front of body as shown, elbows tucked into sides and holding the weights with your palms facing upwards. Now curl your arms upwards until the weights virtually touch the front of your shoulders. Slowly return to the starting position and repeat 16 times for one set.

⑥ Skip or Step for 1 minute

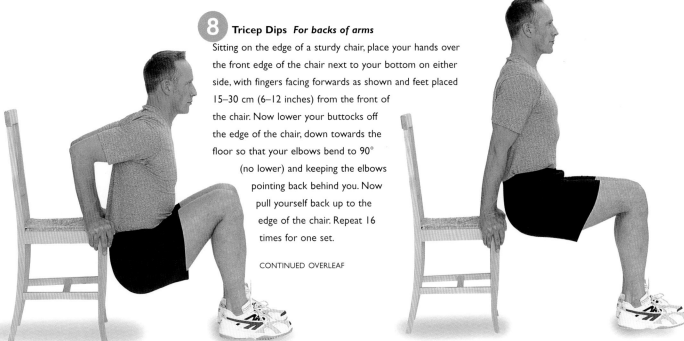

⑧ Tricep Dips *For backs of arms*

Sitting on the edge of a sturdy chair, place your hands over the front edge of the chair next to your bottom on either side, with fingers facing forwards as shown and feet placed 15–30 cm (6–12 inches) from the front of the chair. Now lower your buttocks off the edge of the chair, down towards the floor so that your elbows bend to 90° (no lower) and keeping the elbows pointing back behind you. Now pull yourself back up to the edge of the chair. Repeat 16 times for one set.

CONTINUED OVERLEAF

9 **Skip or Step for 1 minute**

10 **Abs** *For stomach*

Lie on an exercise mat, knees bent, feet flat on floor and legs hip-width apart as shown. Place your hands on your thighs. Using your stomach muscles and breathing out, raise your head a little off the mat, keeping the legs still, and move your hands up the thighs a little as you go. Return smoothly to the starting position. Repeat 16 times for one set.

12 **Press-ups** *For chest and arms*

Kneel on all fours on a mat as shown, spine straight not dipped, stomach tucked in, fingers facing forward and arms shoulder-width apart. Now lower your face towards the floor until a few inches or so above the floor. Slowly return to the starting position and repeat 16 times for one set.

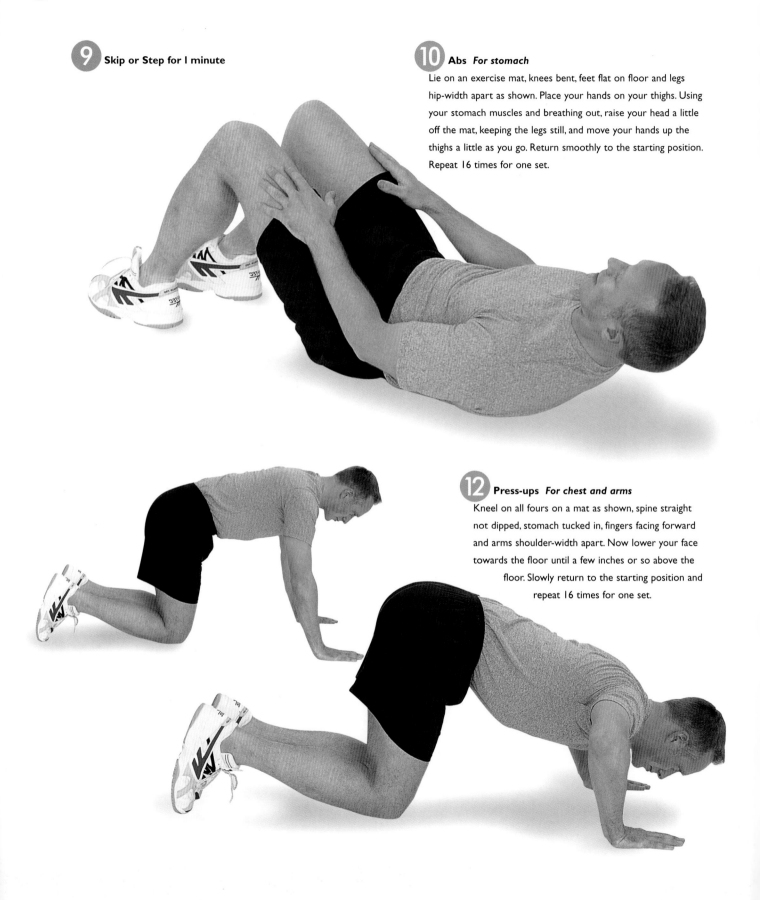

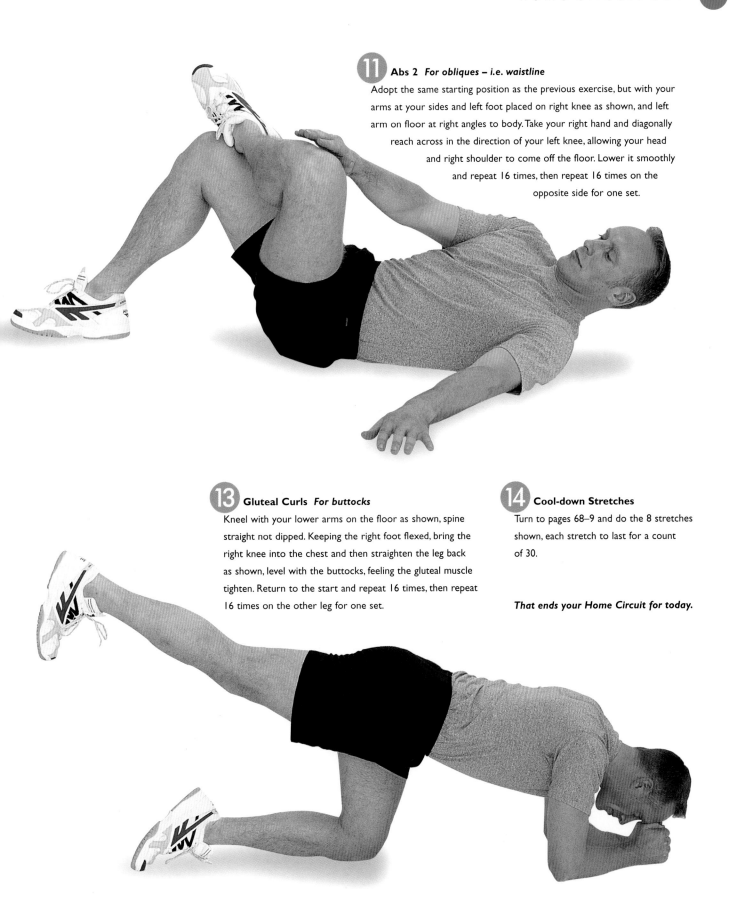

11 Abs 2 *For obliques – i.e. waistline*

Adopt the same starting position as the previous exercise, but with your arms at your sides and left foot placed on right knee as shown, and left arm on floor at right angles to body. Take your right hand and diagonally reach across in the direction of your left knee, allowing your head and right shoulder to come off the floor. Lower it smoothly and repeat 16 times, then repeat 16 times on the opposite side for one set.

13 Gluteal Curls *For buttocks*

Kneel with your lower arms on the floor as shown, spine straight not dipped. Keeping the right foot flexed, bring the right knee into the chest and then straighten the leg back as shown, level with the buttocks, feeling the gluteal muscle tighten. Return to the start and repeat 16 times, then repeat 16 times on the other leg for one set.

14 Cool-down Stretches

Turn to pages 68–9 and do the 8 stretches shown, each stretch to last for a count of 30.

That ends your Home Circuit for today.

HOME CIRCUIT 50+

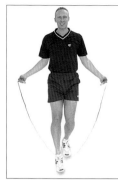

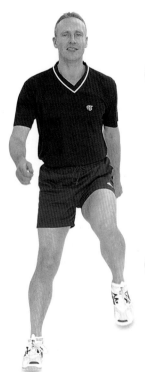

1 **Warm-up:**
March on the spot for 2 minutes, gradually increasing the height you raise your feet from the floor and increasing the amount your arms swing. For the last minute you can march with your legs 40 cm (15 inches) apart if you like.

2 **Warm-up Stretches:**
Do the Quad, Calf and Hamstring Stretches as described on page 68, holding each stretch for a count of 10.

3 **Skip or Step for 2 minutes**
Skip: skip lightly on the spot at a moderate pace, breathing steadily. This will raise your heart-rate. As you get fitter, increase the number of skips you do per minute.

Step: step up and down on a 25-cm (10-inch) step or stair or heavy-weight box (UP right, UP left, DOWN right, DOWN left; then UP left, UP right, DOWN left, DOWN right), stepping down on the floor a few inches from the step each time. Breathe steadily, feel your heart-rate rise.
Check your posture – stomach in, leaning slightly forward.

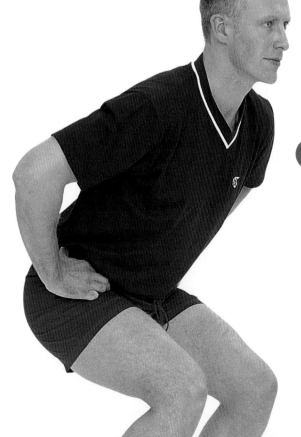

7 **Squats** *For thighs and gluteals*
Stand with the feet hip-width apart and toes pointing forwards, hands on hips, in the correct posture. Now slowly bend the knees without tipping the upper body forwards, until you are 'sitting' with knees bent no more than 90°. Slowly return to the starting position and repeat 16 times for one set; pause for a few seconds, then do one more set.

① CHECK: IS THIS THE RIGHT HOME CIRCUIT FOR YOUR REAL AGE (SEE PAGES 16–17)?

② HAVE YOU READ THE GENERAL INSTRUCTIONS ON PAGE 54 AND THE AT-A-GLANCE CIRCUIT CHART ON PAGE 55?

③ FOLLOW THE NUMBERS AROUND THESE FOUR PAGES FOR DETAILED INSTRUCTIONS ON THE EXERCISES THAT FORM YOUR HOME CIRCUIT.

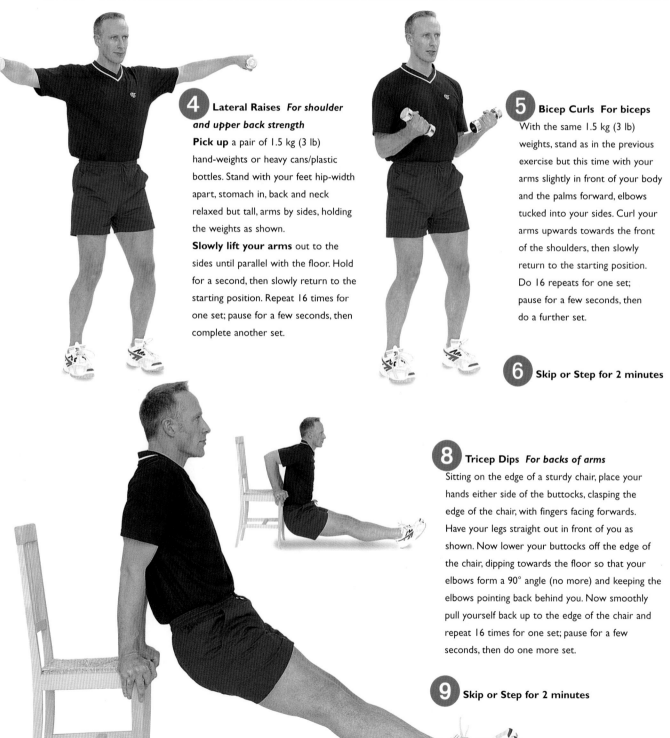

4 **Lateral Raises** *For shoulder and upper back strength*
Pick up a pair of 1.5 kg (3 lb) hand-weights or heavy cans/plastic bottles. Stand with your feet hip-width apart, stomach in, back and neck relaxed but tall, arms by sides, holding the weights as shown.
Slowly lift your arms out to the sides until parallel with the floor. Hold for a second, then slowly return to the starting position. Repeat 16 times for one set; pause for a few seconds, then complete another set.

5 **Bicep Curls** **For biceps**
With the same 1.5 kg (3 lb) weights, stand as in the previous exercise but this time with your arms slightly in front of your body and the palms forward, elbows tucked into your sides. Curl your arms upwards towards the front of the shoulders, then slowly return to the starting position. Do 16 repeats for one set; pause for a few seconds, then do a further set.

6 **Skip or Step for 2 minutes**

8 **Tricep Dips** *For backs of arms*
Sitting on the edge of a sturdy chair, place your hands either side of the buttocks, clasping the edge of the chair, with fingers facing forwards. Have your legs straight out in front of you as shown. Now lower your buttocks off the edge of the chair, dipping towards the floor so that your elbows form a 90° angle (no more) and keeping the elbows pointing back behind you. Now smoothly pull yourself back up to the edge of the chair and repeat 16 times for one set; pause for a few seconds, then do one more set.

9 **Skip or Step for 2 minutes**

CONTINUED OVERLEAF

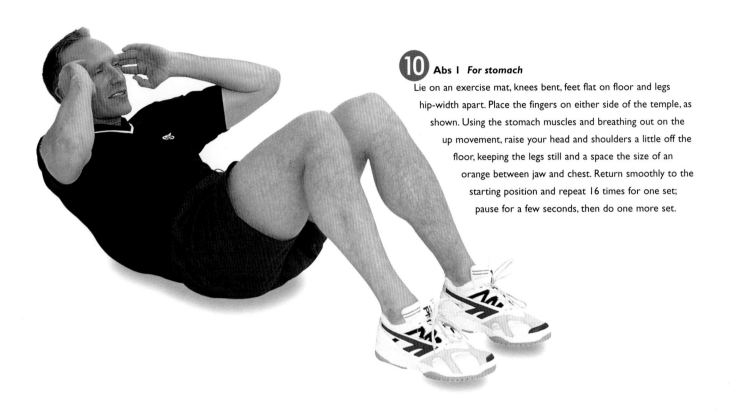

10 **Abs 1** *For stomach*

Lie on an exercise mat, knees bent, feet flat on floor and legs hip-width apart. Place the fingers on either side of the temple, as shown. Using the stomach muscles and breathing out on the up movement, raise your head and shoulders a little off the floor, keeping the legs still and a space the size of an orange between jaw and chest. Return smoothly to the starting position and repeat 16 times for one set; pause for a few seconds, then do one more set.

12 **Press-ups** *For chest and arms*

Kneel on a mat on the floor, supporting the upper body weight with the arms and lower body weight on the knees, with ankles crossed as shown. Keeping your back straight, not dipped, slowly lower the forehead towards the floor, then return to the starting position. Repeat 16 times for one set; pause a few seconds, then do a further set.

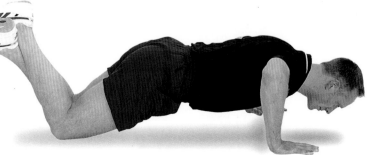

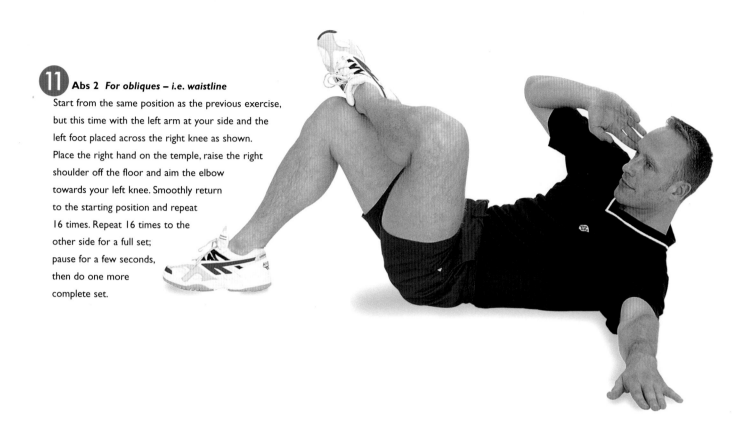

11 **Abs 2** *For obliques – i.e. waistline*

Start from the same position as the previous exercise, but this time with the left arm at your side and the left foot placed across the right knee as shown. Place the right hand on the temple, raise the right shoulder off the floor and aim the elbow towards your left knee. Smoothly return to the starting position and repeat 16 times. Repeat 16 times to the other side for a full set; pause for a few seconds, then do one more complete set.

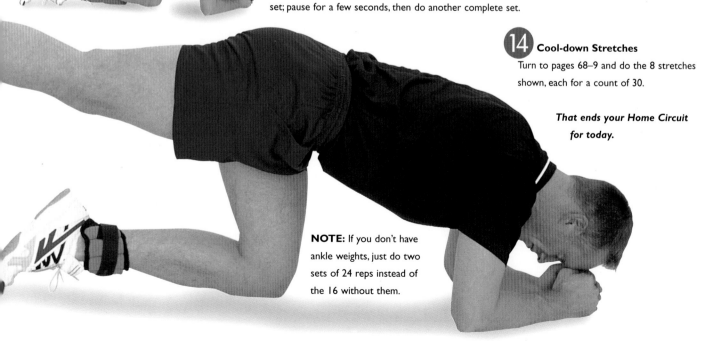

13 **Gluteal Curls** *For gluteals – i.e. buttocks*

Put on a pair of 1-kg (2-lb) ankle weights. Kneel with the lower arms on the floor as shown, spine straight not dipped. Keeping the right foot flexed, bring the right leg into the chest, bending at the knee. Now straighten the leg out as shown, feeling the gluteal muscles on that side tighten. Return to the starting position and repeat 16 times. Repeat 16 times to the other side to complete the set; pause for a few seconds, then do another complete set.

14 **Cool-down Stretches**

Turn to pages 68–9 and do the 8 stretches shown, each for a count of 30.

That ends your Home Circuit for today.

NOTE: If you don't have ankle weights, just do two sets of 24 reps instead of the 16 without them.

HOME CIRCUIT 40+

1 **Warm-up:**
March on the spot for 2 minutes, gradually increasing the height you raise your feet off the floor (to a maximum of a 90° angle at the knees) and gradually pumping your arms harder or doing shoulder presses as shown. For the last minute you can jog lightly if you like, or march with legs wide apart.

2 **Warm-up Stretches:**
Do the Quad, Calf and Hamstring Stretches as described on page 68, holding each stretch for a count of 10.

3 **Skip or Step for 4 minutes**
Skip: skip lightly on the spot, breathing steadily. Gradually increase your skipping pace and vary your steps as you like.
Step: step up and down on to a 25-cm (10-inch) high step, stair or heavy-weight box (UP right, UP left, DOWN right, DOWN left; then UP left, UP right, DOWN left, DOWN right), stepping down on the floor 30 cm (1 foot) or so from the step each time. Breathe steadily, feel your heart-rate rise.
Variation if using a proper step: stand next to one of the short ends of the step, sideways on, with the step to your right side.
Step UP right so that your right leg is just further than halfway across the top of the step. Step UP left. Step DOWN right and DOWN left so that you finish on the opposite end of the step. The next move returns you to the starting position. Shoulder presses can be incorporated as shown.

❶ CHECK: IS THIS THE RIGHT HOME CIRCUIT FOR YOUR REAL AGE (SEE PAGES 16-17)?

❷ HAVE YOU READ THE GENERAL INSTRUCTIONS ON PAGE 54 AND THE AT-A-GLANCE CIRCUIT CHART ON PAGE 55?

❸ FOLLOW THE NUMBERS AROUND THESE FOUR PAGES FOR DETAILED INSTRUCTIONS ON THE EXERCISES THAT FORM YOUR HOME CIRCUIT.

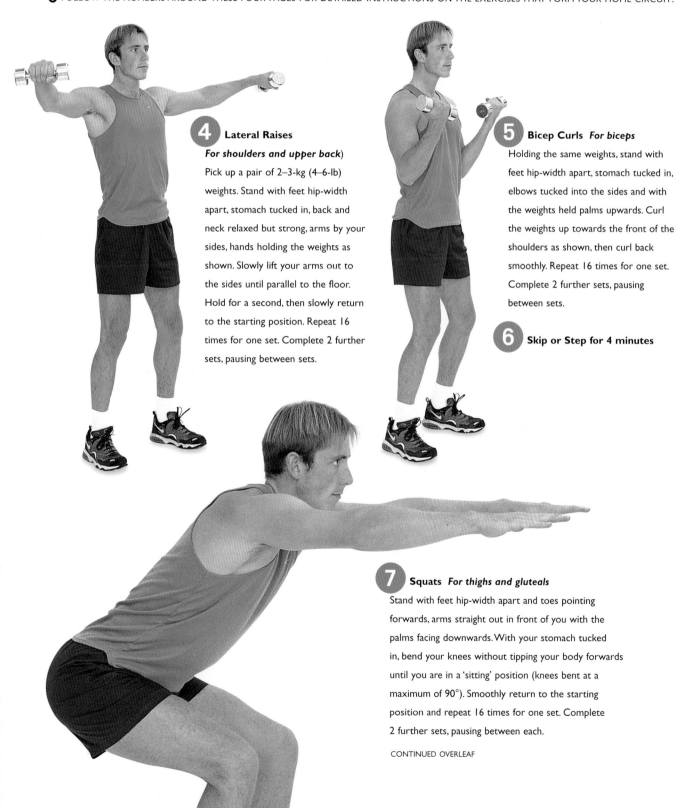

4 Lateral Raises

For shoulders and upper back)
Pick up a pair of 2–3-kg (4–6-lb) weights. Stand with feet hip-width apart, stomach tucked in, back and neck relaxed but strong, arms by your sides, hands holding the weights as shown. Slowly lift your arms out to the sides until parallel to the floor. Hold for a second, then slowly return to the starting position. Repeat 16 times for one set. Complete 2 further sets, pausing between sets.

5 Bicep Curls *For biceps*

Holding the same weights, stand with feet hip-width apart, stomach tucked in, elbows tucked into the sides and with the weights held palms upwards. Curl the weights up towards the front of the shoulders as shown, then curl back smoothly. Repeat 16 times for one set. Complete 2 further sets, pausing between sets.

6 Skip or Step for 4 minutes

7 Squats *For thighs and gluteals*

Stand with feet hip-width apart and toes pointing forwards, arms straight out in front of you with the palms facing downwards. With your stomach tucked in, bend your knees without tipping your body forwards until you are in a 'sitting' position (knees bent at a maximum of 90°). Smoothly return to the starting position and repeat 16 times for one set. Complete 2 further sets, pausing between each.

CONTINUED OVERLEAF

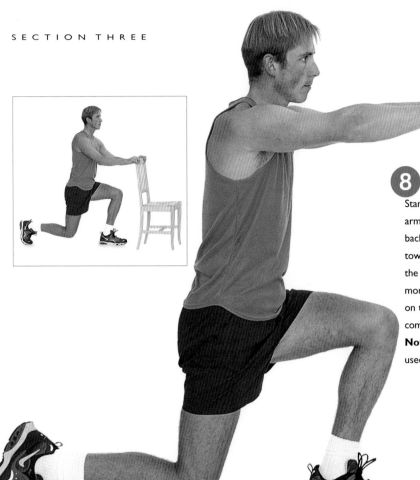

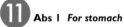

8 Lunges *For gluteals – i.e. buttocks and thighs*

Stand with feet hip-width apart and with good posture, arms out in front as shown. Take one medium pace backwards with your right leg, dropping your right knee towards the floor (but not to touch it and making sure the left foot doesn't move) and bending both knees to no more than 90°. Return to starting position and do 16 reps on the same leg, then 16 reps on the opposite side to complete one set. Do 2 further sets, pausing between each. **Note:** the back of a chair, facing towards you, can be used for support if you like.

11 Abs 1 *For stomach*

Lie on your back on a mat with hands lightly placed on the temples and the knees bent, feet flat on floor. Raise head and shoulders off the floor and, as you do so, bring the bent legs in towards the chest as shown. Lower and repeat 16 times. Complete 2 further sets, pausing between each.

12 Abs 2 *For obliques – i.e. waist*

Lie on your back on a mat with the right leg straight and right arm to the side. Bend the left leg and place the left hand on your left temple as shown. Bring the right knee up towards the chest as shown and, as you do so, raise the head, left arm and left shoulder off the floor and aim towards right knee. Lower and repeat 16 times; repeat 16 times to the other side for complete set. Do 2 further sets, pausing between each.

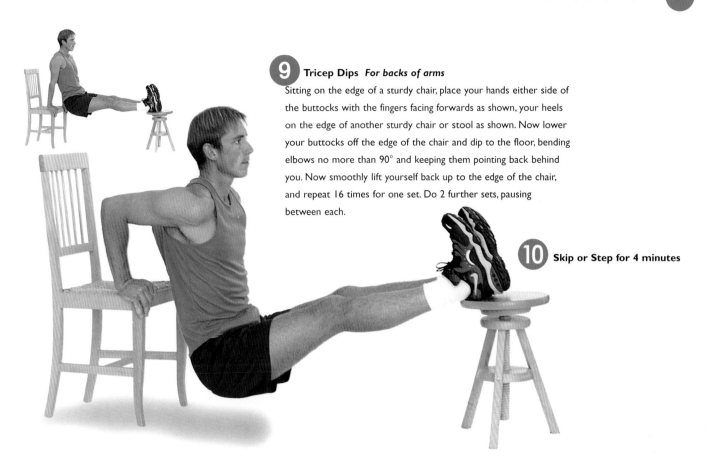

9 **Tricep Dips** *For backs of arms*

Sitting on the edge of a sturdy chair, place your hands either side of the buttocks with the fingers facing forwards as shown, your heels on the edge of another sturdy chair or stool as shown. Now lower your buttocks off the edge of the chair and dip to the floor, bending elbows no more than 90° and keeping them pointing back behind you. Now smoothly lift yourself back up to the edge of the chair, and repeat 16 times for one set. Do 2 further sets, pausing between each.

10 **Skip or Step for 4 minutes**

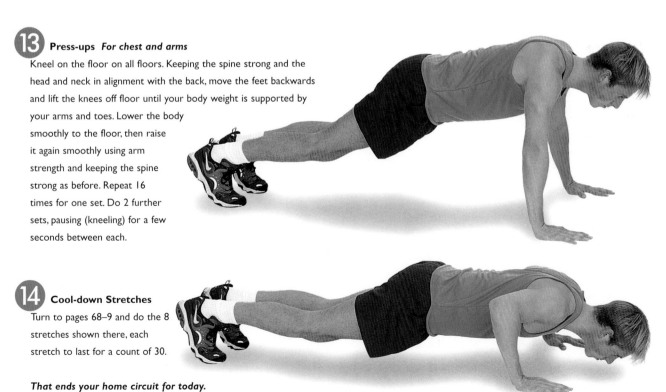

13 **Press-ups** *For chest and arms*

Kneel on the floor on all floors. Keeping the spine strong and the head and neck in alignment with the back, move the feet backwards and lift the knees off floor until your body weight is supported by your arms and toes. Lower the body smoothly to the floor, then raise it again smoothly using arm strength and keeping the spine strong as before. Repeat 16 times for one set. Do 2 further sets, pausing (kneeling) for a few seconds between each.

14 **Cool-down Stretches**

Turn to pages 68–9 and do the 8 stretches shown there, each stretch to last for a count of 30.

That ends your home circuit for today.

COOL-DOWN STRETCHES

❶ USE THE STRETCHES WITHIN YOUR HOME CIRCUIT AS DESCRIBED ON THE PREVIOUS PAGES AND AS DESCRIBED WITHIN THE OUTDOOR EXERCISE PROGRAMME ON THE FOLLOWING PAGES.

❷ WHEN STRETCHING, HOLD THE STRETCH FOR THE DESIGNATED TIME (IN WARM-UP, THIS WILL USUALLY BE A COUNT OF 10, IN COOL-DOWN USUALLY A COUNT OF 30).

❸ IF YOU STRETCH OUT YOUR MAJOR MUSCLES REGULARLY, THEY WILL BECOME MORE FLEXIBLE OVER THE WEEKS, WHICH WILL HELP YOUR POSTURE AND MAY ALLEVIATE ACHES AND PAINS. STRETCHING BEFORE AND AFTER EXERCISE IS IMPORTANT TO HELP MINIMIZE ANY CHANCE OF INJURY, AND IT WILL HELP PREVENT MUSCULAR ACHES THE DAY AFTER EXERCISE.

NOTE: IF YOU FEEL PAIN WHILE STRETCHING, STOP! STRETCHING SHOULD BE TAKEN TO A POINT OF MILD DISCOMFORT, BUT NO MORE.

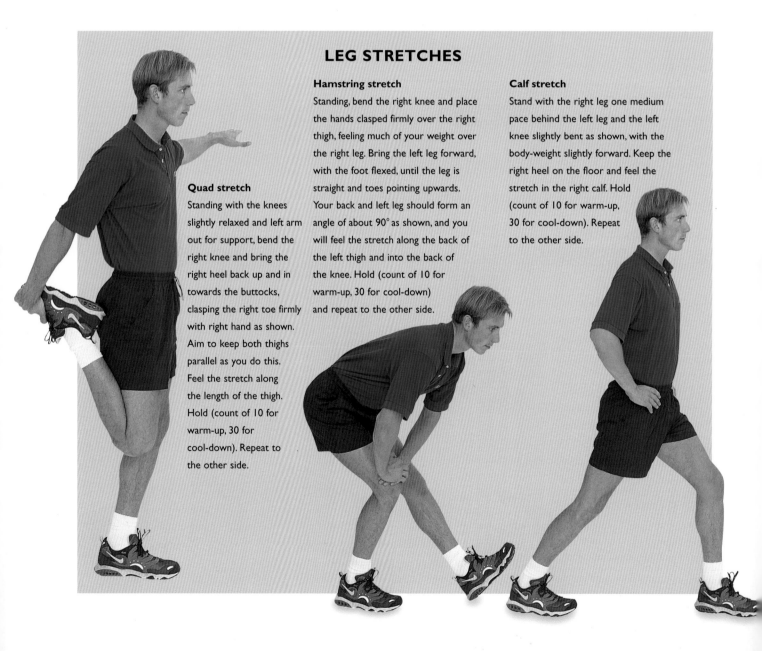

LEG STRETCHES

Hamstring stretch
Standing, bend the right knee and place the hands clasped firmly over the right thigh, feeling much of your weight over the right leg. Bring the left leg forward, with the foot flexed, until the leg is straight and toes pointing upwards. Your back and left leg should form an angle of about 90° as shown, and you will feel the stretch along the back of the left thigh and into the back of the knee. Hold (count of 10 for warm-up, 30 for cool-down) and repeat to the other side.

Calf stretch
Stand with the right leg one medium pace behind the left leg and the left knee slightly bent as shown, with the body-weight slightly forward. Keep the right heel on the floor and feel the stretch in the right calf. Hold (count of 10 for warm-up, 30 for cool-down). Repeat to the other side.

Quad stretch
Standing with the knees slightly relaxed and left arm out for support, bend the right knee and bring the right heel back up and in towards the buttocks, clasping the right toe firmly with right hand as shown. Aim to keep both thighs parallel as you do this. Feel the stretch along the length of the thigh. Hold (count of 10 for warm-up, 30 for cool-down). Repeat to the other side.

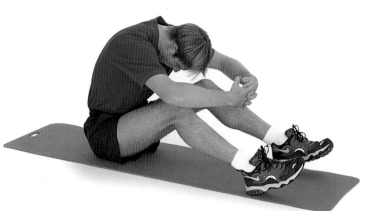

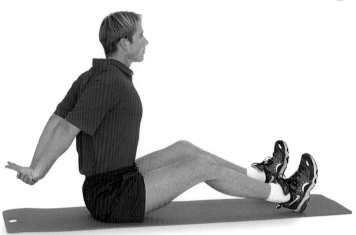

Back Stretch

Sit on a mat on the floor with the legs relaxed, knees slightly bent, stomach tucked in and shoulders relaxed. Now raise your arms into the air, with the hands lightly clasped, and stretch out towards the ceiling (without pushing your head and neck backwards). Now smoothly move the back and arms forward over the lower body as shown, tucking your chin into your chest and feeling the stretch along the spine. Hold for a count of 30.

Chest Stretch

Sit as in the previous stretch. Link your hands behind your back and, keeping your elbows bent, smoothly extend your arms out behind you, pulling your shoulder blades together as you do so and pushing your chest up and out. Feel the stretch across your chest. Hold for a count of 30.

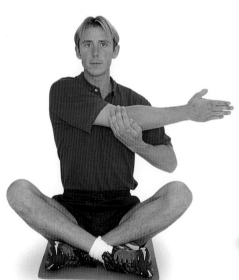

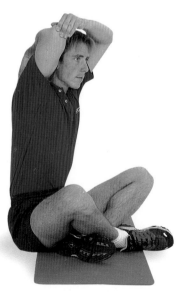

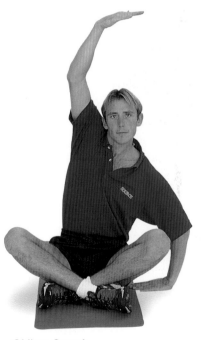

Shoulder Stretch

Sit on the floor with ankles crossed. Bring your right arm across your body at chest level, palm facing inwards. Bring your left arm across and under the right arm and place the left palm on the right arm just above the elbow. Press on the right arm, keeping the right shoulder down, and feel the stretch all over the right shoulder area. Hold for a count of 30, and then repeat to the other side.

Tricep Stretch

In same sitting position as in the previous stretch, lift your right arm above your head and bend your elbow so that your arm forms a right-angle, with the right hand palm-down on your shoulder as shown, hand relaxed. Bring the left hand around and, using the palm, gently press the right arm to feel a stretch all up the triceps (back of arm). Hold for a count of 30, and then repeat to the other side.

Oblique Stretch

In same sitting position again, lift your right arm above your head and support yourself with your left palm on the floor by your left side, fingers pointing in and elbow slightly bent. Bring your right arm over towards the left a little, until you feel a stretch along your right side (the movement is more 'up' than 'across'). Hold for a count of 30, and then repeat to the other side.

OUTDOOR EXERCISE

THE LENGTH OF TIME YOU WILL SPEND ON YOUR OUTDOOR EXERCISE IS THE SAME WHATEVER YOUR REAL AGE, AND BUILDS UP GRADUALLY OVER THE WEEKS ACCORDING TO THE CHART OPPOSITE . DEPENDING ON YOUR REAL AGE, HOWEVER, THERE ARE THREE DIFFERENT WAYS YOU CAN TAKE YOUR OUTDOOR EXERCISE:

In addition to the Home Circuits, throughout the 10-week programme you need to find 3 slots a week for a session of exercise out-of-doors. (The 10-week schedule at the back of the book suggests how this can be organized.) These outdoor sessions will improve your cardiovascular fitness – i.e. the efficiency and strength of your heart, lungs and respiratory system. With a similar programme to this, our four participants improved their resting heart-rate tremendously.

To those of you who are saying 'Aren't the Skip or Step sessions in the Home Circuits enough?', the answer is *no*! Although the Skip or Step sessions will raise your heart-rate for short periods of time, helping to burn off calories and keep your muscles warm, this is not prolonged enough for aerobic (cardiovascular) bene-fit. It is more sustained periods of aerobic activity (a minimum of 20 minutes), carried out regularly, which will help to improve your cardiovascular fitness.

Of course, aerobic activity doesn't *have* to be done out-of-doors – but fresh air is something that most of us have little of these days, so take your cardiovascular exercise outside frequently.

Your aerobic activity will encourage you to breathe deeply, your whole body will be oxygenated and invigorated and, I hope, at the end of every one of your outdoor exercise sessions, you will be more than glad that you made the effort.

GENERAL INSTRUCTIONS ON OUTDOOR EXERCISE

60+

● You will simply walk for the full time described in the chart.

● For the first 3 minutes of your walk, go slowly, gradually building up the pace as you warm up. For the last 3 minutes of your walk, reverse the process.

● After your 3-minute warm-up walking, do the Quad, Calf and Hamstring Stretches on page 68 for 10 seconds each and repeat them after your walk for 30 seconds each.

● Apart from the warming-up and cooling-down period, your walk should be at the briskest pace you can manage without getting too 'puffed'. You should feel your heart working and feel your lungs working, but you shouldn't be stressed. You should stride out, arms swinging moderately vigorously, with your back in good posture and stomach tucked in.

● As the weeks progress you will be able to walk faster and, towards the end of the programme, you will need to take in hill-work in order to continue to progress.

● Alternatively, you may retake the Real Age Assessment and your Real Age may have moved down a band, in which case you can swap to the 50+ Programme.

50+

● For the first 2 weeks you can walk as described for 60+, then swap to cycling: first one session a week, then two a week, and then all three sessions.

● Warm up for the first 3 minutes by cycling slowly or walking with your cycle. After the warm-up, do the Leg Stretches on page 68 for 10 seconds each.

● Cool down for the last 3 minutes by cycling slowly or walking, then repeat the Leg Stretches, this time for 30 seconds each.

● Cycling should be carried out like walking, at the briskest pace you can manage without getting too 'puffed', but so that you can feel your heart and lungs working harder. Later in the programme you can progress by doing more hillwork or by cycling in a higher gear or increasing the weight of your cycle (with weights or panniers).

● Alternatively, you can retake the Real Age test and if your Real Age has moved down a band, you can begin the 40+ Programme.

Note: If you don't want to cycle, you can do the walking programme as described for 60+, but wear ankle weights and do more hillwork right from the start.

40+

● For the first 2 weeks of the programme, walk as described for 60+. Then build in some jogging to your sessions.

● Before you begin a session, warm up and do the Leg Stretches as described for 60+, and cool down at the end, also as described for 60+, repeating the Leg Stretches for 30 seconds each.

Suggested Jog Inclusion:

Week 3: two 1-minute jogging sessions evenly spaced out in the middle of your walk at every session this week.

Week 4: two 2-minute jogging sessions as above.

Week 5: three 2-minute jogging sessions as above.

Week 6: three 3-minute jogging sessions as above.

Week 7: four 3-minute jogging sessions as above.

Week 8 onward: as much jogging instead of walking as you can happily manage without feeling too 'puffed'. By the end of the programme you may be able to jog most of the time at every session. Go at your own pace and use your common sense.

TIME CHART FOR OUTDOOR EXERCISE

Week 1	20 min 3 times a week
Week 2	30 min 3 times a week
Week 3	30 min 3 times a week
Week 4	40 min 3 times a week
Week 5	40 min 3 times a week
Week 6	45 min 3 times a week
Week 7	45 min 3 times a week
Week 8	50 min 3 times a week
Week 9	50 min 3 times a week
Week 10	60 min 3 times a week

Jogging Notes

● It is vital that you have good running shoes and, if you have any joint problems, check with your GP first – and try to choose grass not hard road surfaces to run on.

● Always warm up, stretch, and cool down, then stretch.

● Pay attention to posture as you walk/jog. Keep stomach and buttocks tucked in and head up.

● Wear suitable clothing. Thin layers of clothing are best, as when you get hot you can strip off. (Tie your discarded sweatshirt around your waist or use a small backpack.) You can still go out in the rain – a breathable lightweight waterproof is ideal.

● Wear good-quality shoes suitable for your feet. If you have any foot problems, go to a sports shop and get proper advice on the right footwear for you.

● Take a drink with you. Diluted fruit juice, hypotonic drinks or water are OK.

● Match your route to your ability and try to vary your routes from time to time.

● How do you know it's working? As you get fitter, you will be able to cover more distance in the same time – so you can compare times over the weeks. Last week you passed that gate in 15 minutes, this week you can do it in 12! You also know it's working if you can tackle hills when previously you couldn't, if you can tackle bigger hills more quickly, and so on.

If you have some money to spend, you can invest in a heart-rate monitor which will give you a more accurate picture over the weeks of how your heart-rate is improving (beating stronger but slower) as you walk/cycle/jog, but this isn't strictly necessary.

SPORT FOR ALL

IN ADDITION TO YOUR HOME CIRCUIT AND OUTDOOR EXERCISE, WHY NOT CONSIDER TAKING UP
A FAVOURITE OLD SPORT AGAIN – OR TRYING A NEW ONE?

What is it that men give up on once they turn 40? Not sex, of course, but sport. Spectator sport is fine at any age – doing it, another matter altogether, and this is a huge shame.

Of course, if you're 45 you're not going to be able to match a 25-year-old on the football or rugby pitch, and so pride as well as common sense dictates that there comes a time to bow out of certain arenas gracefully. However, there is plenty of opportunity for participating in sport whatever your age.

The benefits of sport are well documented – not only physical but also social – so here we take a look at the kinds of sport you could be looking at now, with our top 6 analysed for their pros and cons.

**SPORTS TO THINK TWICE
ABOUT OR AVOID:**
rugby, football
squash, hockey
downhill skiing
boxing, martial arts

Swimming

Pros: fairly convenient for most; won't trigger asthma (unlike some sports); supports body-weight, therefore ideal for the elderly, arthritis sufferers and osteoporosis sufferers.

Cons: both public and private pools can get very busy; you get wet; non-weight-bearing exercise doesn't maintain bone density. Ease: suitable for all, but obviously not everyone can swim.

Cost: low.

Health benefits: excellent all round – cardiovascular, strength, tone, suppleness.

Injury risk: very low.

Competitiveness: if you join a local club, they usually have senior age-group competitions.

Tips: it is a good idea to take a course of lessons even if you can swim – technique can always be improved, offering optimum fitness benefit.

Cross-country Skiing

Pros: said to be the best sport for all-round fitness and calorie-burning; ideal if you want to lose weight.

Cons: may have to travel to do it.

Ease: suitable for most if you do a preparatory fitness programme (e.g. the 10-week programme in this book) and build up length/speed gradually.

Cost: moderate to high.
Health benefits: excellent cardiovascular and upper- and lower-body strength exercise.

Injury risk: medium – knee twisting needs to be watched. Competitiveness: cross-country races for varying age groups are organized.

Tips: get fit walking or jogging first; you may like to purchase a ski machine for home use, to help build up the right muscles.

Rowing

Pros: excellent sport for older people, as sitting position reduces chances of joint injury; sociable; good calorie-burner.

Cons: need to be near a river; there may be a waiting-list to join a club; it may not be the sport for you if you have lower-back problems.

Ease: as hard as you want to make it, but not for the very unfit.

Cost: moderate to high.

Health benefits: terrific for cardiovascular and upper-body strength; for bone maintenance.

Injury risk: low.

Competitiveness: plenty of opportunity for competition if you join a club.

Tips: do several weeks of upper-body strength work before beginning — a home rowing machine would be ideal. Otherwise press-ups, lateral raises with weights, single-arm rows, back strength and bicep work.

Tennis

Pros: enjoyable, sociable, competitive.

Cons: not usually aerobic; chance of injury; not an ideal winter sport.

Ease: as hard as you want to make it; not ideal for those with poor spatial awareness, poor sight or slow reactions, though with persistence the sport may improve all of these.

Cost: moderate.

Health benefits: good for mobility (though see Injury risk below); not one of the best sports for cardiovascular fitness unless at advanced level.

Injury risk: moderate (if sensible) to quite high — the twisting and range of movements involved may cause back, shoulder and knee problems, especially in unfit individuals.

Competitiveness: play every game to win — everyone else does!

Tips: do plenty of stretching and strength work before taking up tennis. Warm up thoroughly before every session and cool down with stretches, too.

Golf

Pros: sociable; in fresh air; probably relaxing (though not necessarily).

Cons: nineteenth hole may not be good for waistline; game can be stressful.

Ease: not easy.

Cost: high, unless using municipal course.

Health benefits: will burn quite a few calories in the course of a round, but not particularly good cardiovascular benefit — the walks between holes are not long enough, though if you walk briskly and carry your own equipment this will help.

Injury risk: moderate — back and shoulder problems quite common.

Competitiveness: very.

Tips: reduce risk of injury with regular flexibility and strength work for back and shoulders. Breathe deeply as you walk briskly round the course.

Cricket

Pros: sociable, enjoyable.

Cons: may involve a lot of hanging around rather than playing.

Ease: not easy. Best considered if you used to play; not ideal to take up for the first time in later life.

Cost: low.

Health benefits: won't do much for cardiovascular fitness; stretching for a catch may help flexibility slightly; fresh air good for you; a long match in which you run around a lot will burn up a fair number of calories, so can be good for weight control.

Injury risks: moderate — short bursts of anaerobic activity (e.g. making runs, fielding) may be unsafe for some. Also, cricket balls can be very dangerous missiles!

Competitiveness: very.

Tips: prepare well with flexibility and strength exercises and stamina-building activity, such as brisk walking.

OTHER SPORTS TO CONSIDER:

cross-country running

orienteering

horse riding *if back and joints OK*

netball, basketball

volleyball, table tennis, bowls.

YOUR EXERCISE QUESTIONS ANSWERED

QUESTION 1

I have a bad back – can I still exercise?

Yes you can – with caution. You should check with your GP first, telling him or her what exercise you intend to do. If you want to follow the programme in this book, show it to your GP. While exercising, if you experience discomfort, stop and take a rest or try again another day.

Most research shows that gentle stretching – particularly of the lower back, gluteals and hamstrings – helps prevent back pain, and back and abdominal strengthening exercise also helps. Back extensions – where you lie on the floor on your front, arms at sides, and lift head and shoulders off the floor – are the best exercise for the lower back. When your back gets stronger, you can put hands on the buttocks to increase the difficulty.

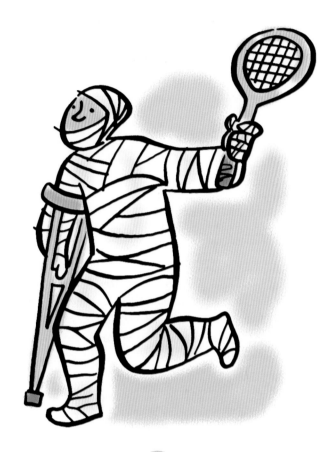

QUESTION 2

I used to have a bad back – what is a safe exercise routine to follow that won't cause a return of the pain?

For cardiovascular (stamina-building) exercise, avoid anything likely to jar the back – such as jogging. Swimming is ideal because the water bears your weight (the crawl is the best stroke for stamina). Walking, wearing decent trainers with cushioned support, is fine.

For strength exercise, the 60+ Programme in this book is an ideal starting point. It is important to work your abdominals, as weak abs place extra stress on the lower back and also produce poor posture, another cause of back pain.

Mobility exercise is very important if you are prone to a bad back – all of the stretches in this book are safe to do if you are sensible. In fact, lower-back pain is often caused by lack of flexibility in the bottom and hamstrings – if these muscles are tight, they tilt the pelvis and this places a strain on the lower back. So do the Gluteal and Hamstring Stretches (page 68) every day.

QUESTION 3

I have arthritis – can I exercise?

Yes – exercise has proved to help arthritis by improving mobility and decreasing stiffness. Exercise helps to maintain or develop the muscles that surround the joints.

QUESTION 4

I have had a heart attack – can I exercise?

Yes – with permission from your doctor. Suitable exercise has been shown to help prevent further heart attacks. How soon you can begin to exercise after a heart attack depends on the individual and, again, is something for your own doctor to decide.

QUESTION 5

I have angina – can I exercise?

Yes – with the consent of your doctor. ANY medical condition needs this consent before you start to exercise. A suitable exercise programme can help improve the efficiency of the heart, lungs and respiratory system, which should help the quality of life for angina sufferers.

QUESTION 6

Is it OK to exercise in late middle years if you have done no exercise for several years?

Yes. It is not only OK, it is important that you do so. It is never too late to start exercising and it will definitely improve the quality of your life – for the rest of your life. If you carry out the Real Age Assessment in this book and begin on the appropriate programme for you, you should have no problems if you're in normal health.

QUESTION 7

What are unsuitable forms of exercise for people at 40, 50 and 60 years of age?

There is no straightforward answer to that, as what exercise is suitable for you at any age depends largely on what you have done in the past, in terms of exercise, and how active you have been. Some 40-year-olds are less fit than other 70-year-olds. When deciding on suitable exercise for you, think of what kind of person you are, what you've done in the past, what things you enjoy, and then use your common sense. For instance, you wouldn't put on your shorts and go for a 10-mile run at any age if you've never run before. Also you shouldn't take up any form of exercise if you have a medical condition, before checking with your GP that it is OK.

While exercising, common sense will dictate if you're doing too much for your current fitness level. If you are out of breath while walking, for instance, then reduce the intensity of the exercise (slow down!) until you feel more comfortable. It is counterproductive to push yourself too hard, too soon, at any age.

QUESTION 8

I have poor mobility and a lot of stiffness and general aches and pains – what is the best way to improve that?

You need to begin a cardiovascular programme, such as the Outdoor Exercise programme in this book (according to your Real Age), which will increase the supply of blood all around the body and will exercise and warm up the major muscles of the body, which can then be stretched. The stretches on pages 68–9 will, then, increase your all-round mobility. Even if your aches and pains are concentrated in one area – say, you particularly suffer from neck and shoulder stiffness – it is important not just to do stretching for that one area. Though you can do extra work on your tighter areas.

QUESTION 9

How quickly can I regain lost fitness after doing nothing for several years?

This depends on various factors, including just how fit you were before you stopped exercising, your exact state of fitness now, and what you do to improve your fitness now. If you were once very fit you will probably find it easier and quicker to regain a good level of fitness than if you have never exercised before. You need to follow a progressive exercise programme, gradually increasing the work you ask your body to do, to gain optimum fitness increases – and you need to do it – regularly. When it comes to exercise, you really do get out what you put in. A 10-week programme like this book should, for most people (whether or not they have exercised much in the past), give good results – better posture, better flexibility, firmer muscles, increased strength and stamina, and a general sense of well-being.

QUESTION 10

How quickly will I see results in my body shape?

If you follow the programme in this book, after 10 weeks you will certainly notice a difference in the way you look. This may partly be due to your posture being better. Your stomach will also be flatter and your general outline improved.

looking good

The message you give when you look good is positive.

The way you look matters more than you may admit. Just because you're a man that's no reason to feel vain every time you look in a mirror, or impossibly egocentric if you wash your hair every day or care about clothes.

Yes, it is true, a truly vain man is not a pretty sight (even if he thinks he is) and is often disliked equally by both sexes. However, looking after your looks and using all means at your disposal to keep yourself looking great every day is *not* vanity: it is being flattering to the people you are with and kind to yourself.

Looks matter, primarily because they are the most important and immediate way of showing *who* you are. How easy it is with a practised eye to glance at a stranger and sum up how he feels about himself and the world.

If you look good, you will have more self-confidence, and justifiably so, because others will have more confidence in you, too. The message you give when you look good is positive. If you look good, you will also look years younger. Conversely, if your looks are letting you down, you are more likely to be lacking in self-confidence and looking *older* than your years.

In this section we look at all the areas of the 'outer you' not covered by our diet and fitness sections – hair, balding, greyness and beards . . . skin problems and cosmetics. However, probably the greatest impact upon your looks can be made by what clothes you wear, so we discuss your wardrobe, both formal and informal, and help you decide whether it needs updating, assisting you to find the fine line between looking modern and going 'over the top'. We tell you what women really like and hate their men to wear. Top stylist, Ceril Campbell, also makes-over our four participants to suit their lifestyles – a feature that will give you plenty of ideas for your own revamp.

It's never too late to change – just make sure these changes are the *right* ones . . .

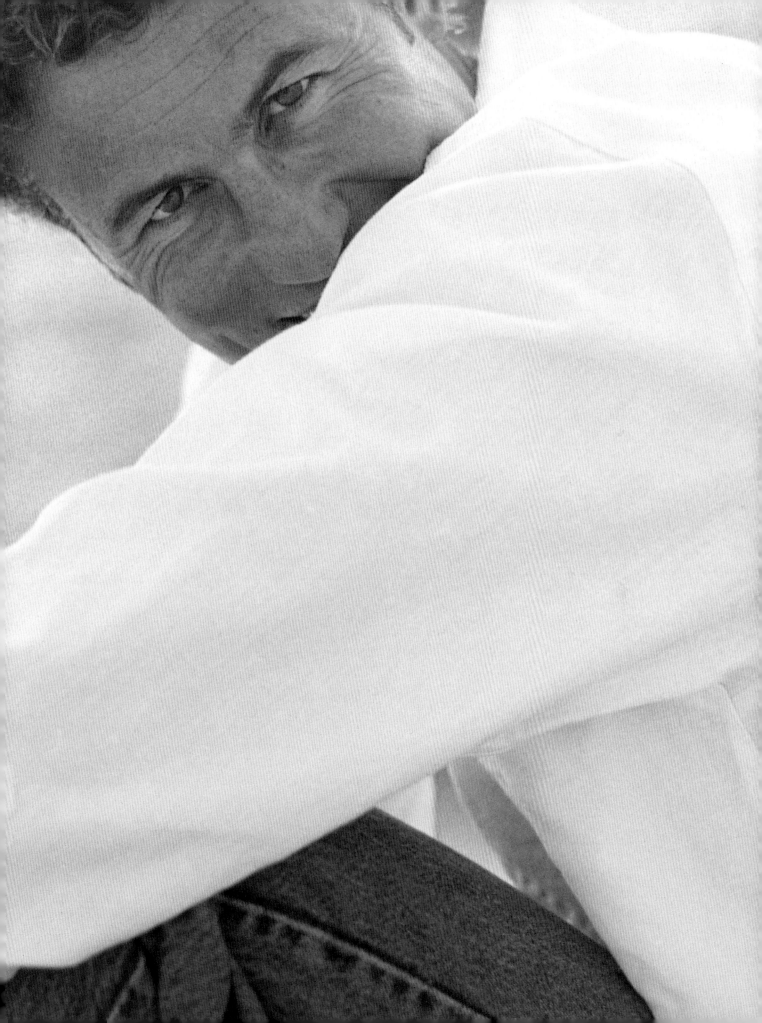

HELP FOR HAIR

YOUR HAIR HAS JUST AS STRONG AN IMPACT UPON OTHERS AS YOUR LOOKS, YOUR PERSONALITY OR YOUR CLOTHES. THE WRONG HAIRSTYLE CAN ADD ON YEARS, THE RIGHT ONE TAKE OFF A DECADE, SO TAKE A FRESH LOOK AT YOUR OWN 'CROWNING GLORY', WITH THE HELP OF OUR TIPS HERE.

FOR YOUTHFUL
NOT LAUGHABLE
LOOKS

AVOID

● hair all one length all over

● hair longer than collar length

● tied back hair

GO FOR

● light layering/movement to add body and shape

● the best hairdresser you can find

● A shape of cut that suits your face

If you're trying to hang on to your youth – and your youthful good looks – the worst mistake you can make is to keep your hair as you had it then. Few things look worse than an older, greying, wrinkled man with long locks, a pony tail or a perm. Apart from anything else, if you haven't changed your style in years, it dates you straight away.

You also need to consider the texture of your hair, which may have changed since you were a young man. Hair may get coarser and drier with age, in which case very short cuts are best. It may also get thinner and 'floppier', in which case, again, a shorter cut will give it more 'lift' and help you look younger.

Whatever your hair type, there are numerous terrific products in the shops these days to help you manage it in style. Long gone are the days of a dab of Brylcreem. Shampoos and conditioners are formulated to suit every conceivable hair type, so pick the right one for you. Dry coarse hair needs plenty of moisture and a weekly deep conditioner will help.

Styling mousses, gels, lotions, creams and sprays abound - all are designed to be left in your hair, not rinsed out. Many (mousses, leave-in conditioners, anti-frizz products) are applied to damp hair, which you then dry and style with a dryer; others (gels, creams, some sprays) can be used after your style is dried, or when you are leaving it to dry naturally

– they will then add texture, volume, moisture or hold.

Which one to pick? A mousse tends to thicken the hair (good for fine or thinning hair); gel firms it and keeps it in place very well (good for fine, flyaway hair). Creams tend to add shine and moisture (good for dry, coarse hair). Lotions and sprays aid styling (e.g. when used with a hairdryer, they may help to straighten the appearance of hair) or may add holding power or a little volume or shine or conditioning – read the labels.

Depending upon your hair-type, you then need the best cut you can get – a good cut will go with the hair texture and volume and complement the natural way it grows. Most importantly, it will suit your head and face shape and point up your best features.

You should be much more concerned about what suits *you*, than what may or may not be in fashion right now. As a general rule, older men tend to look younger if their hair is 'lightened' by layering. Few older men can get away with a centre parting – it elongates the face and nose. A long face and nose should go with a side parting and some kind of fringe.

Beards and moustaches should be treated with extreme caution (at any age, but more so the older you get). A greying beard can add years to you and is to be avoided at all costs, whereas if your

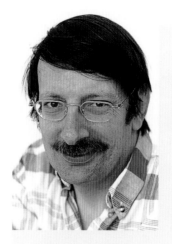

BEFORE

Chris Hall, on his own admission, hadn't paid any attention to his hairstyle for years. 'Do you like your current style?' we asked him. 'I don't know,' he said. 'I never give it any thought.' What about the moustache? 'Same,' he said. 'It's just there.'

stubble is not grey, a little bit of stubble can slim your face down and make you look younger.

A very short moustache can look good if you have a wide gap between nose and top lip or a long face. Be warned, however, most women detest moustaches and there is nothing more of a turn-off than a milk, beer or food-covered moustache. A moustache also rarely makes you look younger – the reverse is usually true.

Grey hair is nothing to be ashamed of. Certainly don't consider dyeing it – greying hair can look chic and elegant and the colour actually suits most men; whereas, if you dye it is immediately apparent and will elicit more snide comments than compliments. It's the male version of mutton dressed as lamb.

Baldness is the main cause of follicular complaint amongst middle-aged men the world over. It is one of the few areas within the battle of the sexes where women win hands down – 90% more men than women go bald. You know what to blame – hormones again.

You must surely know by now that what you don't do if you're going bald is to try to hide the bald patch by growing long strands over it. What you *do* do is get a good, short haircut – and stop worrying. In a recent poll of what women find unsexy in men, baldness came way down the list of dislikes.

AFTER

We persuaded Chris that a change would be an improvement and put him in the hands of stylist Calvin at MichaelJohn in London's West End. Calvin removed the 'flat helmet' effect by trimming the overall length of the hair and then layering through the front, which also opened up Chris's face and helped balance the shape of the head. Next Calvin trimmed the sideburns, which we all agreed looked too old-fashioned. The style was finished by blow-drying and applying a little light grooming cream to help keep Chris's fine hair from flopping. Calvin then cut Chris's moustache back to a short stubble – we removed the rest of it with a razor. As we had suspected, Chris looked much younger (and more good-looking!) without his moustache.

His verdict? Modesty forbade him to say very much – but he looked incredibly pleased!

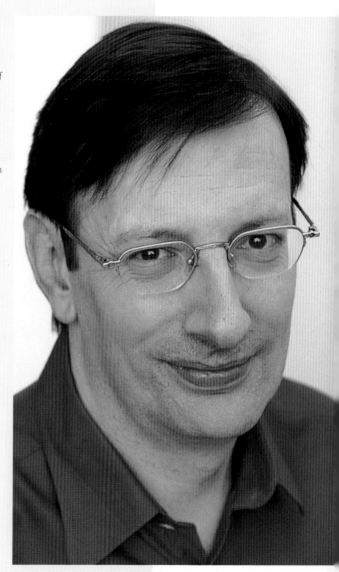

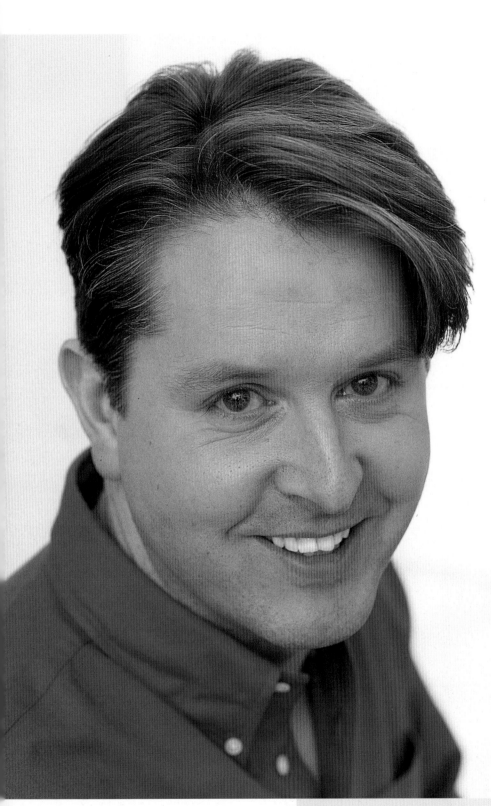

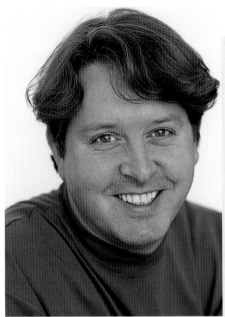

BEFORE

Chris Hampson had, for some years, been determinedly hanging on to the large mane of hair flopping foppishly over his forehead (the 'Hugh Grant' look, though he hates to hear those words). 'I think it makes me look younger', he said. However, Chris was impressed with the idea of having his hair restyled by London's top male salon and allowed stylist Vincent a free rein. Vincent felt that the 'flop' was just too heavy and that it was, in fact, dragging Chris's looks down.

AFTER

'I've kept the general spirit of the style, but got rid of much of the weight and interpreted it in a much lighter way,' said Vincent. 'Chris's hair was all one length on top and at the sides, and it was tending to bush out and looked untidy quickly, too.'

Vincent layered through the top and sides of the hair, while keeping a similar length. When he blow-dried, he applied a smoothing cream to add staying power and shine – bringing out pale-brown lights in Chris's healthy head of hair.

Chris's verdict? 'Yes, it's excellent; the condition is good and I agree that, no, I don't look older at all!'

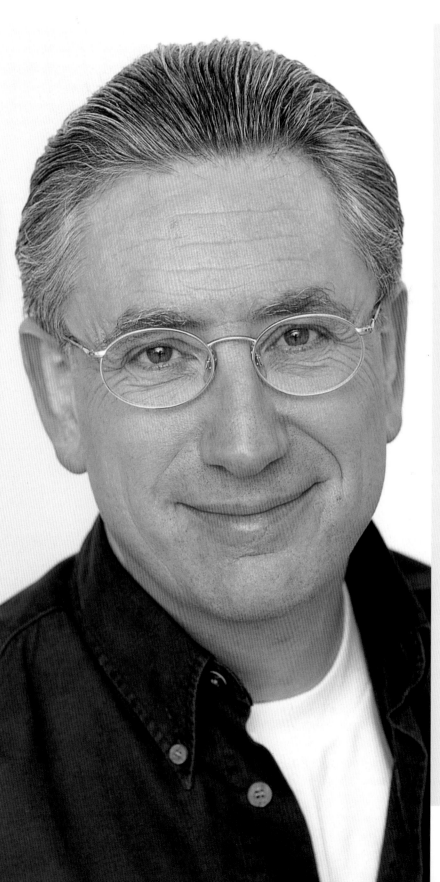

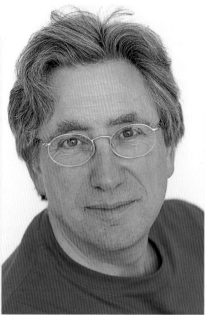

BEFORE

When we met Roger he had been growing his hair longer for some time and it was very Peter Sellers circa 1970. Unlike many men in their 50s, Roger is lucky to have plenty of hair and, if anything, it borders on being almost too thick to be manageable. Roger's hair has greyed to the 'salt and pepper' look – which we all agreed suited him very well.

AFTER

Calvin felt that a sleek, smooth look would suit suave Roger and bring him bang up-to-date. 'I am going to trim the overall length a little and take most of the weight off all over to show off the shape of Roger's head, which is good. I am also going to take the hair mostly back off his forehead, to accentuate his excellent face shape and good features, and if he wants to, he can bring a few strands down for a more casual look.'

Calvin advised Roger to apply a small amount of grooming gel or cream from the palm of his hand every day after washing the hair to keep it smooth and looking in top condition. Roger will still look good when this style grows a centimetre or so longer – as long as he keeps the layered movement.

SAVING YOUR SKIN

WHY IS IT THAT WOMEN SPEND BILLIONS OF POUNDS A YEAR ON SKIN-CARE, TRYING TO PREVENT OR REVERSE THE AGEING PROCESS, AND YET MEN DON'T? IF YOU WANT TO LOOK YOUNGER, IT PAYS TO TAKE A LEAF OUT OF THE FEMALE BOOK. HERE'S MY GUIDE TO THE TIPS AND PRODUCTS THAT WILL HELP YOU.

WHAT SKIN-SAVING MEASURES TO TAKE?

When skin ages, if you leave it to its own devices, various changes take place: it dries out; it loses its elasticity (which can be minimized by regular facial exercise to keep the underlying muscle tone good); and it becomes more wrinkled and coarse.

The ageing process is speeded up by exposure to the sun (a lifetime in the sun – estimated at 50,000 hours – will increase wrinkling by over three times) and by smoking – heavy smokers are nearly five times more likely to be wrinkled than non-smokers of the same age.

Obviously, staying out of the sun (or using a sun-block every day, e.g. Body Glove's waterproof sun-block, 0171 792 3134) and not smoking are the two best ideas. These days, however, all the signs of skin-ageing can be minimized with a few lotions and potions used daily.

First a word about which brands to use. There are several ranges designed especially for men e.g. Aramis has produced the new U-Turn Age-Defying Formula for men, which is widely available, and the French company Nickel for Men (0541 505000) has a good selection. Boots and Nivea also have men's items; but if you stick to the male-only brands you will have much less choice than if you are prepared to buy those aimed at women too. Male and female brands differ in packaging (men's versions in 'manly' bottles!) and

perfume content (if any – obviously men don't often want to go round smelling of lilies, or whatever) but sometimes in very little else. Basically, the male and female skin are the same, so cosmetics should be unisex (though some cosmetic scientists will tell you that, as men's skin is thicker than women's, products for men can be stronger).

MOISTURISERS

Many of the signs of ageing can be helped with a daily moisturiser that you can smooth on after your shave (see Shaving Balms, right) and again at bedtime, unless you are using a different night cream (see below). The trick here is to know the buzzwords and pick one that suits your skin, as well as one that will have the most effect. Also bear in mind that dry skin needs water – get an Evian spray (from Boots) and use it on your face before moisturising and regularly on your face during the day, especially if you are in a dry atmosphere.

● AHAs are fruit acids which, when formulated in a moisturiser, will have a mild or stronger exfoliating effect similar to a chemical facial peel, leaving the skin smoother, more refined and pinker. Some skins can be sensitive to these. Many moisturisers are on the market containing AHAs, and this will be stated on the pack.

● Retinol is vitamin A, which it is claimed (though more scientific trials need to be done) – affects the

deeper layers of the skin, stimulating cells to grow and building collagen to improve elasticity, improving the look of lines and wrinkles. Diminish, by Estée Lauder is one widely available new brand and skin-care company RoC makes a range of retinol-containing creams in their Actif Pur range, which is also widely available and not too hard on the pocket.

● Antioxidants (see page 27) are appearing more and more often in face formulas; they are said to help neutralize the free radicals formed from pollution, smoking, sun damage and the ageing process, and thus help prevent the signs of ageing. I would say that Vitamin E is the most popular antioxidant (e.g. the widely available L'Oréal Futur-E), and pure vitamin E is perhaps the one skin product that I personally would always use above everything else. I use natural vitamin E capsules (e.g. Seven Seas) broken into my palm and spread on the face before bed, as you get a bigger 'dose' this way.

NIGHT CREAMS

The dividing line between a night cream and a day cream is often thin – packs don't always give guidance and some products can be used during the day and at night. A good rule-of-thumb is if the product is still visible, or very shiny, on the skin after smoothing it in well, it should best be used at night. Be warned, some night creams are just too heavy and may worsen the appearance of open pores.

SOOTHERS / SHAVING BALMS

Some beauty experts say that men have younger, smoother skin than women of the same age because, in shaving daily, they remove the top layer or skin and encourage smooth new skin to form.

If your skin tends to get easily irritated, instead of the usual shaving mousses try Professional Shave by Dermalogica (0800 591818) which contains skin-calming essential oils and silicones.

After shaving, instead of slap-ping on the same old after-shave you've been using for 20 years, try one of the new soothing balms, such as Post-Shave Healer by Clinique (widely available). A good balm will feel cooling, soothing and moisturising. The herbal extract aloe vera is a good soother and is contained in several balms and moisturising lotions, e.g. Aloe Vera Gel by Face Stockholm (0171 734 1234).

TONERS / ASTRINGENTS

Men don't really need these – if you have open pores, a slap with ice-cold water will do as much good. Toners don't actually close pores at all, and if you're shaving every day you won't need astringents as much as soothers.

MASKS/EXFOLIANTS REJUVENATORS

Once a week or so it is quite a good idea to use a 'treatment' product to help your skin along. Face masks which you smooth on, avoiding the eyes, mouth and nostrils, and leave for several minutes – can be moisturising (e.g. Stuck in the Mud by Philosophy, 0870 607 7060),

and/or purifying and/or refining, (e.g. widely available Masque Controle by Lancôme) and/or 'rejuvenating' (e.g. Morning Mask by WU). Decide what you want to achieve and buy one of the hundreds of products available to suit. You can also try an exfoliant that you smooth into your skin using fingertips and rinse off straight away (e.g. widely available Never a Dull Moment by Origins). These are, however, best avoided if your skin is sensitive.

SKIN TONE

After 40, your naturally good skin colour may start to fade. Best advice is to take regular exercise, which will give you a good colour and refine pores.

Very pale skin can also benefit from a light smoothing of fake tan – if you haven't tried one for years, forget the orange, multi-streaked effect, things have moved on since then. Clarins is a good one. Though make-up for men is going to take a while longer to catch on in a big way, you could get away with a tinted moisturis-er, such as Crème Lumière by Ultima 11 (from Boots) which comes in four colours and con-tains light-reflecting particles that minimize fine lines. If you're too frightened to use it during the day, you'll definitely get away with it in the evening.

For over-florid skin tone, first try cutting down on alcohol, if you drink a lot, and you can also try a green-tinted moisturiser. Avoid AHA creams and exfolia-tors, both of which may make the redness worse.

Area by area

EYES

There are many eye creams on the market claiming to be anti-wrinkle, anti-dark circles, and so on. You may just prefer to use your ordinary face creams instead of these. There are also gels for helping to reduce bags and puffiness. Cold tea bags and cucumber slices also work well, as does aerobic exercise, because baggy eyes are often the result of poor circulation (for the same rea-son your bags will always be less noticeable in the evening than when you wake up in the morning).

Red eye whites can be brightened almost immediately by adding a few drops of Murine (widely available) to each eye – but don't use it too often. You can also improve the brightness of your eyes with enough sleep, little alcohol, a good diet that includes plenty of vitamin C, a healthy liver, regular bowel function and regular exercise.

BODY SKIN

Facial moisturisers tend to be more expensive than body lotions, so buy a separate one for smooth-ing out dry patches on hands, elbows, knees, feet, and so on. Widely available E45 cream is inexpensive and good, or try Boots 12-Hour Hydrating Body Lotion with vitamin E.

HANDS

Dry hands are a dead give-away of your age, so use a rich hand-cream (E45) every time your hands have been in water and at night. Brown age spots (liver spots) on hands are the bane of many older men. Several products claim to reduce or remove them. Try RoC Actif Pur Anti-Age Hand Treatment (widely available) or Decleor Whitening Powder Complex (0171 262 0403). Also remember to look after your nails – eat a good diet, and

when using your hand-cream smooth it well in around the cuti-cles. There's also nothing wrong with a regular professional manicure if you can afford it.

TEETH

Yellowing, stained teeth really don't look good. For white teeth, don't smoke or drink strong tea or coffee or red wine. There are many tooth-whitening pastes on the market, but some may damage the teeth due to their metal-particle content, and the deter-gents that they may contain have even been linked with mouth ulcers. Mouthwashes have also been linked with oral cancers.

Look out for Yotuel, a paste that contains the natural cleaning enzyme papain, if you want white teeth. Alternatively, if you can afford it, you can have professional tooth-whitening (e.g. a company such as Dentics).

FEET

Men don't look after their feet! I know this now for certain, having weighed many men in their bare feet when auditioning for this book and having seen, all too frequently, every kind of neglect possible. I don't know how you all walk around on feet that bad!

Feet take all your weight every day, stay encased in stuffy, hot, airless shoes all day and you never think about them ever unless they hurt or you get athlete's foot or a verruca. Wash them daily, moisturise them, cut their nails to a sensible length regularly and use a deodorizing anti-bacterial foot powder. Give them stylish comfortable shoes (more than one pair) and then you will look younger, because if your feet are happy, you are happy. So will your partner be. Men with bad feet are a turn-off!

CLOTHES WISE

IF YOU WANT TO SHED THE YEARS, IT'S ABOUT TIME FOR SOME DRASTIC RETHINKING OF YOUR WARDROBE.
WE HAVE ENLISTED THE HELP OF TOP STYLIST CERIL CAMPBELL TO GIVE YOU – AND OUR PARTICIPANTS –
PLENTY OF GOOD ADVICE OVER THE NEXT 10 PAGES.

**TOP 10 GIVE-AWAYS
OF YOUR AGE
(ALL BEST AVOIDED!)**

- White socks
  unless at the gym

- Shell suits

- Short shorts

- Leather blouson jackets

- V-neck sleeveless sweaters

- Cowboy boots

- Cummerbunds with your
  dinner jacket

- Brushed check cotton shirts,
  like Grandpa's

- Braces

- Knitted ties
  (old-fashioned sort)

WARDROBE SHOOTING

The average man spends a quarter of what the average woman does on clothes. When quizzed on this anomaly, men often say that male fashion hardly changes over the years and they can therefore get away with the same old items. However, men's style does change, in subtle ways. And you change too – your colouring, your looks, your personality. What suited you years ago won't suit you now.

Even the least sartorial of men will probably find a few things in the wardrobe that are worth keeping, to mix and match with some new items. Though don't be tempted to hang on to the '70s loon pants and kipper ties – yes, the '70s are back but not that back. If you are sure you will look good in clothes that owe much to the past –

buy the new millennium versions. Before you ransack your cupboards for anything worth keeping, first you need to update yourself on new looks.

Plan of action

❶ Look in the pages ahead and see what we did for our four participants, which will give you some ideas and starting points.

❷ Make a list of things that you think suit you and another of things that don't. Try different colours up against your skin and hair and see which ones work and which don't. If your hair has changed colour in recent years, your best colours may also have changed. Think about what materials suit you – as we get older we often need better quality. Generally speaking, shine and glitz and loud patterns are out; understated is in. Think about your body shape and what styles suit you (see Body shapes and styles right).

❸ Buy some current men's magazines for more ideas on up-to-the-minute looks. The Ralph Lauren adverts in men's magazines are ideal examples of relaxed current dressing, but *don't* be a slave to current trends – just make a note of the best bits (and then only the bits that are suitable for your lifestyle). Try to keep an open mind but not lose a cool head. If you've worn nothing but shell suits or baggy cords for leisure and three-piece suits for work for the last 20 years you may be in for a surprise.

❹ Now go through your own wardrobe and see what you have that will fit in with a more flattering, up-to-date image for yourself. Don't be tempted to hang on to stuff that is grotty or cheap or ill-fitting, or that you have hardly ever worn.

❺ Write a list of a capsule wardrobe that you need (for many men this will be 2 suits, 3 shirts, 6 ties, 2 sweaters, 2 pairs of casual trousers and 2 pairs of shoes) and then go round the shops trying on items that fit in with all the previous criteria. This is the worst bit for many men. If you can afford it, then, get a personal shopper. Alternatively, go for mail order – no longer just full of naff stuff, most catalogues have designer ranges at very good prices.

Body shapes and styles

SHORT:
Go for fitted styles – baggy clothes will swamp you – and shorter-length jackets – long ones will shorten your legs even more. Outfits co-ordinated all in one colour produce an elongating effect, as do vertical lines, such as pin stripes. Don't wear double-breasted suits or turn-ups on your trousers.

TALL:
You can carry off most styles if tall and slim. Wear your height with pride! If you do want to appear less tall, wear a top in a different colour from the trousers to make a break in your line, and wear turn-ups.

WIDE:
Go for dark single-breasted suits with pale shirts. Buttons in a contrasting colour can detract attention from width. Narrow belts. Waistcoats. Avoid blouson jackets, thick-knit jumpers, anything with an elasticated waist. Avoid double breasts.

POT BELLY:
Avoid anything tight over it. Avoid 'builder's bottom' with jeans. Avoid straining tight shirts and wear well-cut dark-coloured jackets to broaden the shoulders and detract from the girth.

FACES, NECKS AND COLLARS:
Match your face and neck to your shirt collars and make yourself look better!
Long thin face: choose a big collar but not too wide.
Wide, round face: choose a longer, thinner collar.
Long neck: choose a high-cut collar.
Short neck: choose a lower-cut collar.

GOING PEAR-SHAPED

LAWYER CHRIS HALL WAS, ON HIS OWN ADMISSION, COMPLETELY SARTORIALLY CHALLENGED.
CERIL CAMPBELL HELPS TURN HIM INTO A STYLISH SOLICITOR.

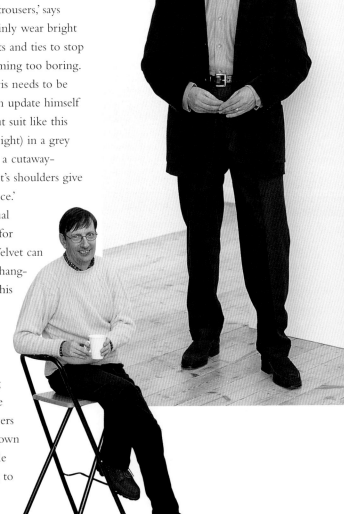

When Chris Hall wrote in to us asking to join the 10-week project, he admitted that he had 'no visual sense of style'. When we met him, we had to admit that his summary was accurate! Chris had perfected the just-got-out-of-bed, harassed look and had a huge pile of casual clothes circa the '80s that had been 'doing a turn' for perhaps longer than is wise – the shirt and past-their-best chinos in this photo are typical.

'Apart from anything else they are highly unflattering to his figure, which is – unusually for a male – rather pear-shaped,' says Ceril. Even though Chris has lost his surplus weight and shaped up, he still carries most of his weight in the lower half and has quite narrow, sloping shoulders. The pale baggy trousers (belted with a dark belt, which just draws attention to the middle) and the baggy shirt tucked in simply make him look wider around the middle.

'A better casual look for Chris would be a pair of dark trousers with a slimmer line, and a plain sweater (right). He should avoid sweaters with raglan sleeves – seams that go diagonally from neck to armpit, and go for ones in which the seam runs from shoulder to armpit,' says Ceril, 'So broadening the shoulders.'

Chris finds most men's clothes boring and enjoys bright colours, so we put him in yellow – also a good colour to cheer you up.

Chris's work clothes had traditionally been rather out-of-date suits. 'Chris isn't clothes-confident enough for bright colour in suits or even trousers,' says Ceril, 'But he can certainly wear bright clear colours in his shirts and ties to stop his work suits from seeming too boring. However, for work Chris needs to be fairly traditional and can update himself perfectly with a well-cut suit like this one from Hackett (far right) in a grey chalk stripe, worn with a cutaway-collared shirt. The jacket's shoulders give him a broader appearance.'

For a smart-but-casual occasion, Chris was all for velvet, but says Ceril, 'Velvet can rather smack of hippie hang-over. Chris should try this soft lightly tailored moleskin jacket for a more modern velvety feel (above right). We'll team it with something Chris would never have thought of – grey trousers and beige shirt with brown suede loafers. The whole outfit is quite flattering to the figure and looks much more relaxed without a tie.

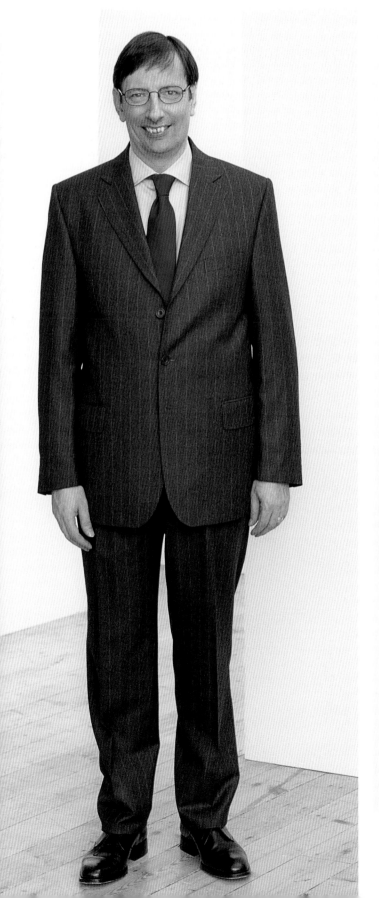

GIRLS DO MAKE PASSES . . .

The majority of men over 40 wear glasses at least some of the time, and many men aren't wearing a pair that flatters them. Change your glasses every year or two – even have two or more pairs so that you can pick the ones that go best with what you are wearing. Chris models a selection of glasses for us and Ceril comments on them.

❶ Chris's own glasses – suit him well but aren't making much of a style statement.

❷ Alain Mikli frames are too rectangular, too strong in colour and too dominant for Chris's fairly small and fairly angular face.

❸ These Armani glasses are good – modern, not too dominant as tortoiseshell is not too dark, and softer on his face, with a good stylish frame shape. They make him look younger.

❹ From DKNY, these glasses are excellent for Chris – they make him look serious and authoritative for his job, but not too much so, and the shape really suits his features.

❺ These round Armani frames are just too round and too much of a contrast with Chris's angular face shape.

❻ From Silhouette – the frame is too large for his face, the bridge too strong, too deep and old-fashioned. The colour is also wrong for his skin-tone.

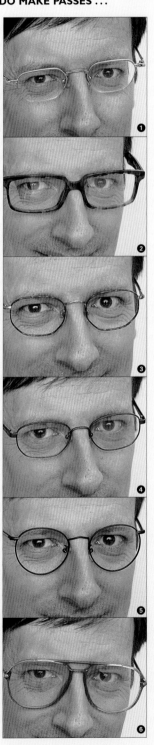

FINDING THE RIGHT CUT

HAVING LOST A STONE, CHRIS WAS EAGER FOR SOME ADVICE ON WHAT TO WEAR.

A busy architect with his own partnership, Chris has to tread a fine line between looking smart and not 'stuffy'. Having slowly put on weight over the past decade, he had not felt inclined to buy lots of clothes in that time, 'you always intend to lose the weight and *then* buy the clothes'.

At 6 feet 2 inches and broad with a capital B (think rugby scrum-half and you have it!), Chris found that the suit label that fitted him best was Boss. Says Ceril, 'When choosing a new suit, try on various designers because the cuts vary tremendously. Once you find a basic cut that suits you, it is worth sticking with that designer as, generally speaking, his or her suits will always look well on you'.

This blue/grey Boss suit (far right) is perfect, with nothing more than a black casual shirt underneath for the office or going out. Swap the casual shirt for a more formal shirt and tie, and Chris has his outfit for meeting clients or for dinner dates (inset). Says Ceril, 'Chris needs a fairly big collar as he is a big man. And if he chooses a button-down style he will look trendier'.

With his home, business and family commitments, Chris keeps an eye on the wallet but was pleasantly surprised to find that this suit was less expensive than he thought. 'You can get a very decent quality suit for £3-400, and these days you can get one that looks perfectly good for £150,' says Ceril. 'If you remember the golden rules – choose a dark plain colour, make sure that it hangs well on the shoulders and that the fabric is good, and then accessorize well – people will think you have on a much more expensive suit than you really have. If you can't afford top-of-the-range designer suits, go for their more reasonably priced diffusion ranges, sold mail-order or in the high street.'

For weekend or evenings at home, Chris loved these black moleskin trousers (right) that made him look even slimmer than he now is. Ceril teamed them with a woollen sweater from Burton's Menswear, cleverly striped horizontally across the chest to accentuate Chris's manly chest and showing off his newly slim stomach. As an alternative to the dark hues that suit Chris so well, we teamed the moleskins with a blue button-down shirt from Hackett (see page 132).

Now he is fit, Chris has been able to take up football again and was keen to try on some modern tracksuits. This one (far right) is from High and Mighty. Warm and comfortable, it will take him to the sports field or the gym.

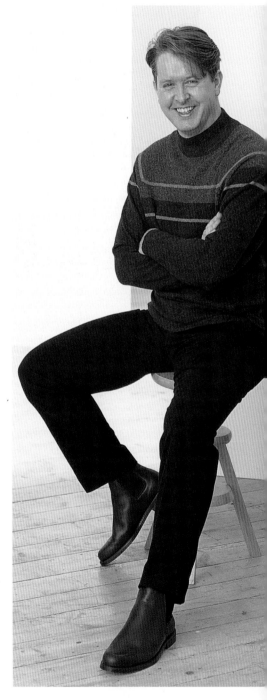

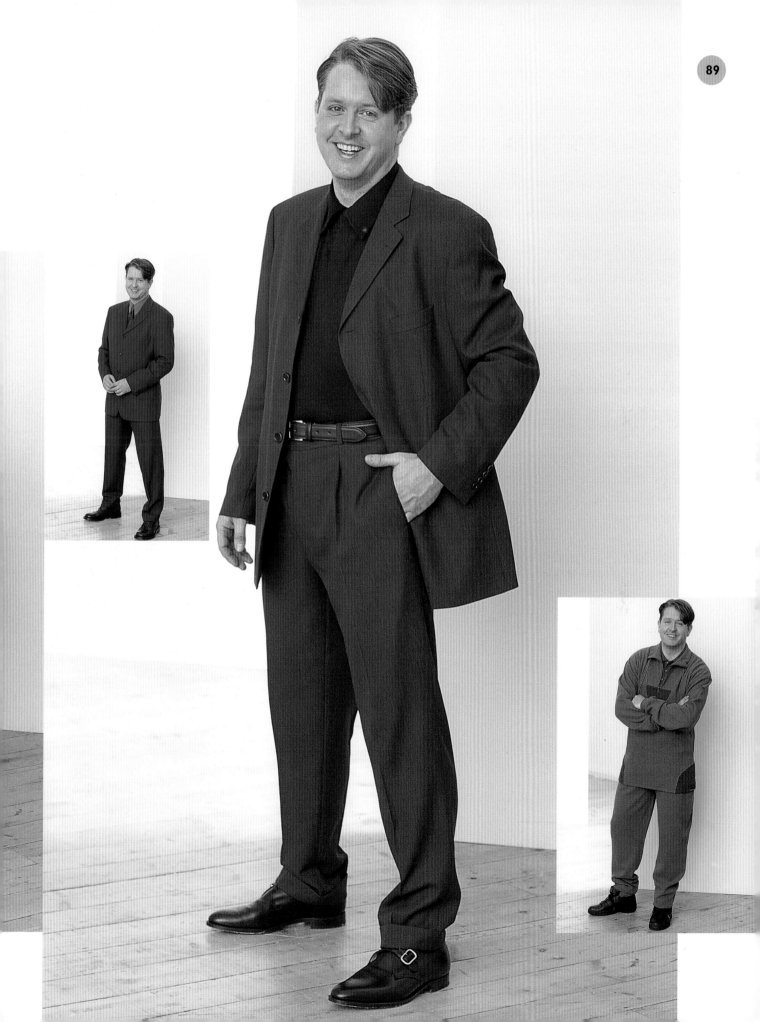

LIFE AFTER BLUE JEANS

A BUSY, BUSY, CAR-BOUND WORK-LIFE, A FULL SOCIAL LIFE AND A PENCHANT FOR BLUE JEANS – WHAT ADVICE COULD CERIL GIVE TO NOEL?

Noel has dressed ultra casually all his adult life. He used to sing in a band that was once a support-ing act to the Kinks and, with his laid-back personality, still likes to wear jeans . . . and more jeans. 'I have nine pairs at home!' he admits, most of them blue, and this is a typical Noel outfit. 'I pull a pair on in the mornings with a polo or T-shirt and that's it!'

Says Ceril, 'If you're in your 40s and 50s you have to be careful about jeans, otherwise you do look like a leftover from the '60s or '70s. Particularly avoid wearing them with your old cow-boy boots and leather jacket. However, you can wear jeans if they are a pair with a modern shape and *not* bleached-out. Today's best denim colour is dark-blue, much more up-to-date. The current shape is straight but wider, not close fitting to the leg – but I hesitate to give advice on that as fashions in jeans change quite quickly!

'I think Noel should try the late '90s alternatives to denim – moleskin casuals, or chinos.' Here (centre) Noel wears navy moleskins from Marks & Spencer,

which show off his neat new waist really well, teamed with a Ralph Lauren button-down shirt that gives the ensemble a real touch of class. Noel has a Hackett plain wool sweater to put on when it is chilly and the brown Timberland deck shoes and brown leather belt complete the look. 'I don't feel too dressed up in this,' says Noel, 'And I do like the moleskins a lot; they are even more comfortable than jeans.'

For a slightly more smart casual look, Noel could wear a blazer – this one (right) is superbly soft 100% cashmere, teamed with chinos and a white T-shirt. How to wear a blazer without looking like a refugee from the Army and Navy club!

Noel doesn't wear suits a lot, but did like the idea of purchasing a new one when he saw himself in this Boss suit (far right), which Ceril teamed with a dark purple shirt and tie for a completely modern look. 'Don't feel you have to wear pale or bright shirts and ties,' she says. 'This twist looks quite dramatic and suits Noel well. Men with grey hair can

look fabulous in dark grey, charcoal and black.' Noel also looked great in the striped dark-grey suit with orange shirt and tie that he's wearing on page 134 – not at all traditional, but definitely not 'mutton dressed as lamb' either.

'Some men in their middle years just can't get away with trendy looks at all, but Noel has the type of personality that means he can be a bit bold.'

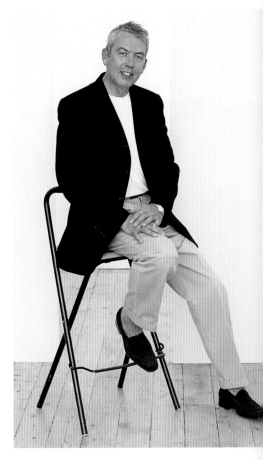

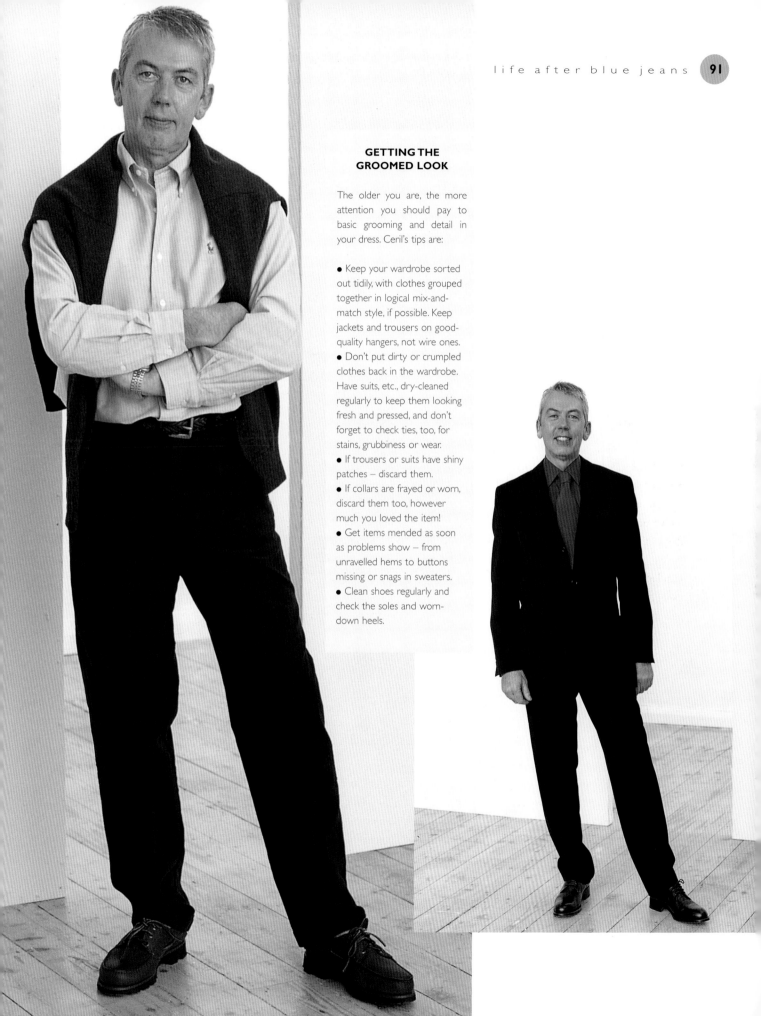

GETTING THE GROOMED LOOK

The older you are, the more attention you should pay to basic grooming and detail in your dress. Ceril's tips are:

● Keep your wardrobe sorted out tidily, with clothes grouped together in logical mix-and-match style, if possible. Keep jackets and trousers on good-quality hangers, not wire ones.
● Don't put dirty or crumpled clothes back in the wardrobe. Have suits, etc., dry-cleaned regularly to keep them looking fresh and pressed, and don't forget to check ties, too, for stains, grubbiness or wear.
● If trousers or suits have shiny patches – discard them.
● If collars are frayed or worn, discard them too, however much you loved the item!
● Get items mended as soon as problems show – from unravelled hems to buttons missing or snags in sweaters.
● Clean shoes regularly and check the soles and worn-down heels.

REDISCOVERING THE SUIT

A NEW HOME AND A NEW JOB FOR ROGER – WHAT HE NEEDED WAS A NEW LOOK, TOO.

The same week we brought Roger into the studio to photograph him in some new clothes, he started a new job – his first time working for anyone other than himself in sixteen years!

'I have to look smart to the office, of course, though it needn't be too formal a look. I haven't bought a new suit in ages – the last time I did, I went out and bought five all the same style at the same time, then put on weight and needless to say hardly wore those suits at all! I would like to look smart but not too traditional.' Roger's own outfit (left), which he wore to our studio, is not flattering to him at all and has seen better days.

'I am also moving to the country shortly and need some advice on what to wear, apart from quilted waist-coats and baggy cords!'

For working days, Ceril first put Roger in a grey Boss suit (right) the cut of which was flattering – broadening his shoulders and slimming the waistline, which is still slightly larger than Roger would like despite having lost four inches off it in 10 weeks!

Says Ceril, 'A good tip is to make

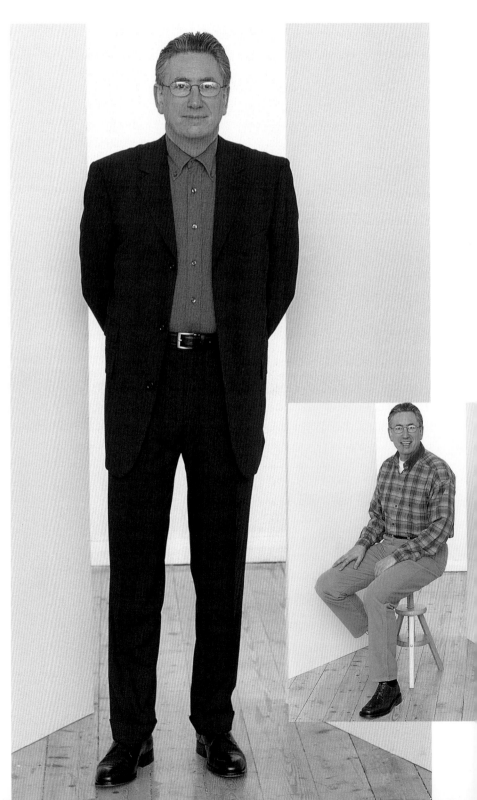

sure that the shoulders of your jacket are at least as wide as your hips.'

She added a grey button-down shirt, which looked very smart worn without a tie. 'Of course you can add a tie if you want to – and make it as bright as you like,' says Ceril, 'Or choose a bright shirt and dark tie as we did in the photo on page 135.'

An alternative smart outfit for working days could be separates – a good jacket such as this one (right) from Hackett in grey tweed with blue windowpane check matched with some grey flannel trousers and given a lift with a pink cut-away-collar shirt and pink-and-blue spot tie. Pink is one of Roger's good colours – he suits clear blues and pinks best of all.

For the country, Ceril suggested this pink tartan cotton shirt with a trendy cord collar, teamed with a pair of camel moleskins (left) – warm and very comfortable. 'There are plenty of modern alternatives to traditional Viyella check shirts (such as the one Roger wore in his photo 10 weeks ago, see page 9) and cord trousers. Moleskins for colder weather and chinos or brown denims for summer will look good on people of any age. Another tip for looking smart in the country in cold weather is to layer your clothes, rather than wearing a huge baggy thick knit jumper. Don't be afraid to wear a plain T-shirt under your shirt – it looks very nice.'

SHOE SENSE

'Men don't pay enough attention to their footwear!' says Ceril. 'They let themselves down by old-fashioned, scuffed, dirty, worn shoes when a new well-kept pair could transform an outfit.'

● For formal wear, go for a good-quality lace-up for day – brogue types are substantial and always look good – and a more elegant slip-on, perhaps, for evening or in summer.

● For casual wear, nothing beats a loafer style.

● Stick with black, shades of brown or dark tan. Avoid burgundy and trendy colours – they are horrible! Avoid fussy shoes, such as ornate plaited-leather uppers and huge fancy buckles. Less is more when it comes to foot decoration – but do go for a shoe that looks substantial enough with your outfit. Particularly, if you are a big man, wear a big shoe.

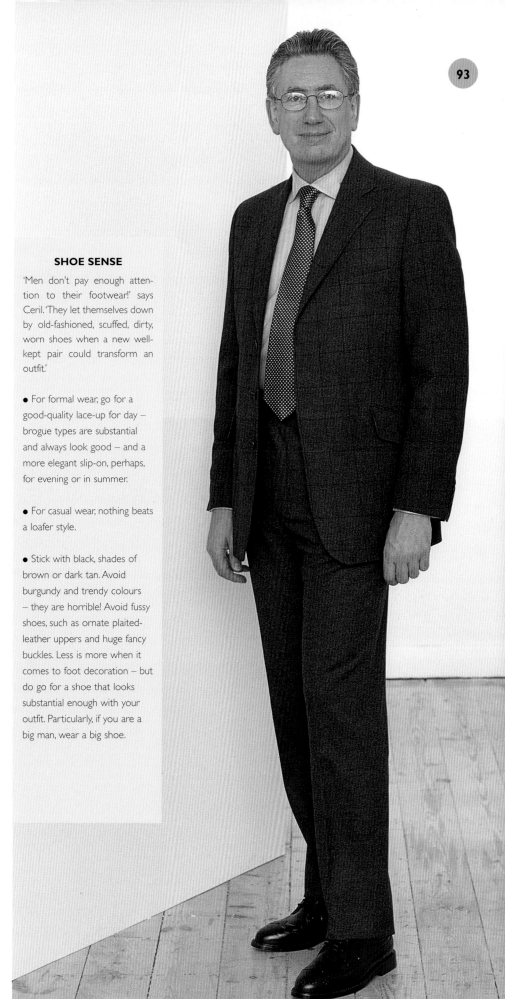

sex &
relationships

Good sex and loving relationships can keep you young – and that's a fact.

more sex for longer life

Men who maintain an active sex life into old age act younger and appear younger than those who don't – and research has shown that men with live-in partners are happier and live longer than those without. Conversely, men who live on their own, with little or no sex, are more miserable and have shorter lives. That is why I have included a section on sex and relationships in this book.

For this important section, I have called upon the help of one of the UK's top sex and relationship counsellors, Phillip Hodson. Phillip comes with a long list of credentials – he is a Fellow of the British Association for Counselling, a Trustee of the Impotence Association, a UKRC-registered Independent Counsellor and a member of the British Association of Sexual and Marital Therapists. He also comes with a vast wealth of experience, of course – he has written eight books of his own, has been 'agony uncle' for five UK newspapers and nine magazines and on radio (currently with Jimmy Young on Radio 2), and has his own private psychotherapy and sex therapy practice in London. Lastly, he has huge amounts of common sense and humour. So, apart from the small quiz on pages 104–5, the rest of the words in this section are Phillip's. He will be explaining why sex keeps you young, how to improve your sex drive and performance in mid-life and later, and how to keep interest going in a long-term relationship.

Many men in mid-life are going through a period of change, or at least considering change. Phillip looks at the pros and cons of splitting with a long-term partner and guides you through the minefield of forming new relationships, offering pertinent advice on how to attract new lovers – and what turns them off.

You will find out that 10 weeks *is* long enough to sort out what's good and what's not so good about your personal life and to begin to take steps towards making any changes that may be necessary.

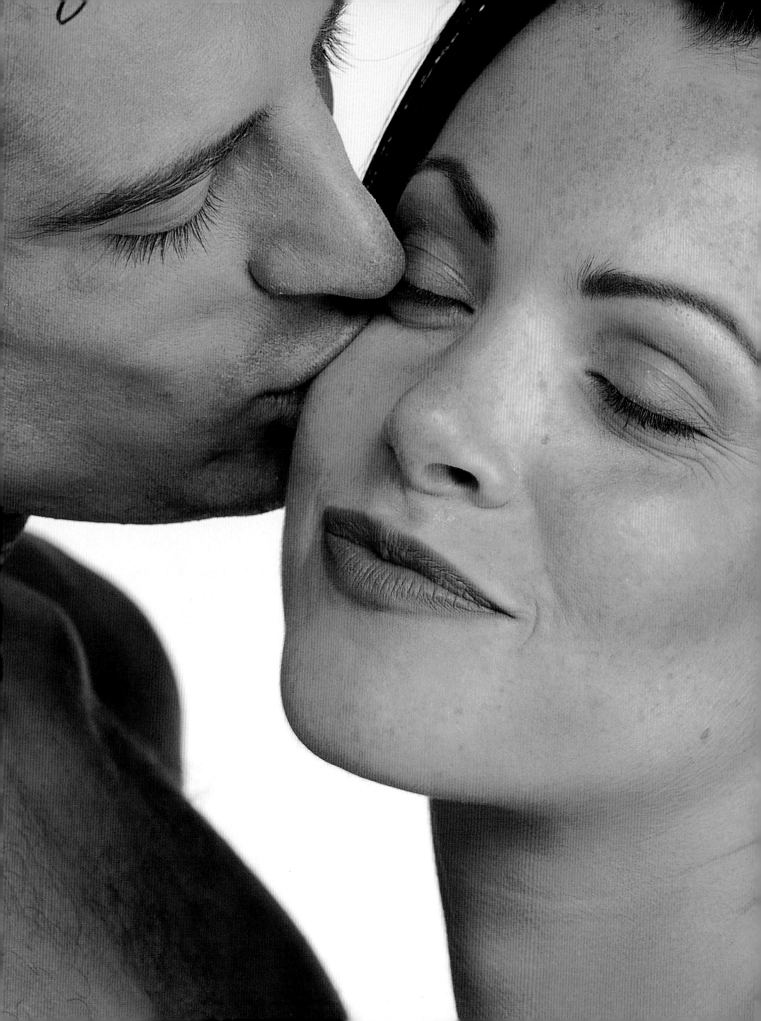

YOUR TOP 10 QUESTIONS ON SEX

QUESTION 1

Why does sex keep you young?

A good sex life is almost bound to keep you young. Recent health statistics show that a satisfying love life actually extends the male life-span and helps you to good health and well-being. (And for the same reasons, will help you feel younger – JW.) Here are the major benefits:

● Sex is first-class exercise. First, you need to be fit enough to be able to walk up a set of stairs without running out of breath. Then again, it's quite important to be able to move your major joints freely. So supple-ness and stamina both count.

   It also burns off plenty of calories. Sex three times weekly can burn an extra 8,000 calories a year. A decade with little or no sex translates into 80,000 unused calories – that's a stone and a half of fat, one big paunch!

● It's good for the prostate gland by ejecting potentially harmful substances.

● Sex increases your respiration rate, which sends more blood round the body to nourish and warm all the internal organs. Speeded-up blood flow throughout the body removes pressure from the brain that could otherwise be harmful.

● The rush of noradrenaline at climax helps reduce snoring. Regular snorers are at higher risk of heart trouble.

● Sex relieves stress without medication or cost. Orgasm reduces tension, especially of the neck and shoulders.

● Sex boosts levels of DHEA, a hormone that increases powers of concentration and may boost the immune system.

● Sex can make you a more affectionate and considerate partner by releasing the hormone oxytocin during orgasm. People with high levels of this hormone initiate more cuddles than those with lower levels.

● Sex is one of the most powerful painkillers known to the human body, because of the endorphins and enkephalins (opiate-like substances) released into the brain after climax.

● The touch of others is vital for keeping you young. It has been proven that children who are raised without affection and physical contact may develop brain damage, and that elderly people with pets to stroke live healthier longer lives than those who don't. The psychologist Dr Eric Berne wrote, 'Touch deprivation may even call forth a transient psychosis or give rise to temporary mental disturbance. If the brain stem is not sufficiently stimulated, degenerative changes in the nerve cells may follow . . . stimulus-hunger has the same relationship to survival of the human organism as food-hunger.' Or, to sum it up: 'If you are not stroked, your spinal cord will shrivel up.'

   There's also a huge youthfulness 'gain' from giving and receiving sexual satisfaction. A good lover plays mind games and has fun – he's not always serious, with a head full of facts and figures – and this produces the perfect antidote to stress. A good lover remains open to new ideas and he experiments. He's a part-time psychologist, able to read his partner's moods.

   So it's easy to see why a lover is literally staving off mortality. Doctors researching aspects of middle age have now worked out a formula which suggests that good sex reduces the risk of premature death by as much as 36% per 100 orgasms.

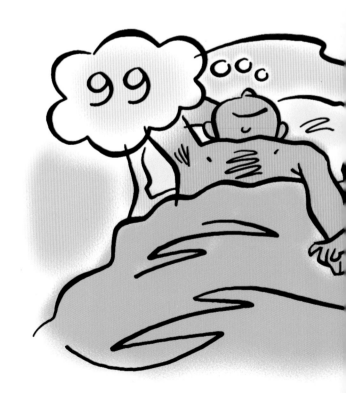

QUESTION 2

How much sex is normal in the middle years for men?

Sexually, men hit their peak at 20, so it's not surprising that middle age sees some decline. Most men over 35 discover that work, age and family take their toll. Hormones play a part. There's a long-term fall in available testosterone throughout adulthood. However, some men respond paradoxically. One 'menopausal' male suddenly began making love to his wife six times a day! Rates of lovemaking are also affected by other factors. For instance, some individuals are naturally very highly sexed. It's normal for a few men to want sex constantly, and also for a few men to want sex never.

A 'honeymoon' effect raises rates of lovemaking whenever a new affair or relationship develops, and a 'boredom factor' reduces them in long-term relationships, as does the increased risk of impotence. However, most middle-aged men appear to make love about once a week on average, while masturbation is known to continue throughout adult life.

The biggest factor affecting sex rates isn't the decline in male hormones, however, it's the failure to keep investing time, trouble and variety into what happens in the bedroom – and that is under personal control.

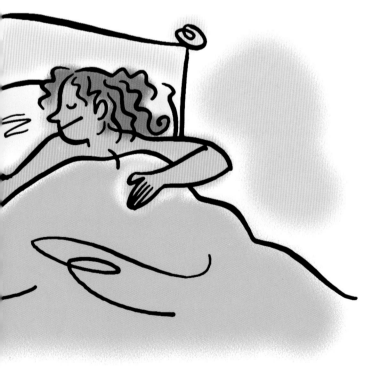

QUESTION 3

How much sex is normal in the later years for men?

After 60, in the so-called 'third age', sexual health really depends on over-all physical health. Or, as the author of *The Joy of Sex*, Dr Alex Comfort, once put it: 'The same things that stop you from riding a bicycle stop you from having sex – only it's later for sex.' Rates of sexual activity after 60 tend to fall to two to three times a month, although most men remain fertile until death.

One health problem tends to dominate all proceedings and that is the curse of impotence. By the age of 75, well over a third of men will be suffering from symptoms of impotence unless treated with one of the new remedies. Again, however, there is a real difference between the amount of sex a man has and his potential enjoyment. Very often various psychological factors, such as bad grumpy marriages and low levels of self-confidence, prevent men from reaching their full erotic potential. Obviously, quality matters too, but lack of quantity also influences the outcome.

A well-tried medical principle suggests that if you don't use a system in the body then it will decay. So the more sex you *do* have, the more you *can* have.

QUESTION 4

How can I improve my sex drive without Viagra?

Viagra is not an aphrodisiac, because you will still have to be sexually stimulated by foreplay for it to work. Better and more varied foreplay, however, is nearly always the best way to improve sexual drive. Sexual satisfaction also depends on feeling there is a strong drive for sex. A University of Michigan study found men in their 70s were just as happy with their sex lives as men in their 30s so long as drive and erections remained intact – regardless of whether they got enough sex. It's knowing you want it that counts. And the best way to increase your drive? Sexual satisfaction is a simple equation – how closely does what you get out of sex measure up to what you expected? If your expectation of your performance and partner is sky-high, you'll kill satisfaction.

Bear in mind the 'Rule of Twos'. Of 10 sex acts, two may be wonderful, two rotten, while six may be mediocre. Having boring sex stops you wanting sex. If you ate Beluga caviar every day you'd soon get sick of it.

QUESTION 5

Is Viagra a good idea?

Viagra is a clever product but, like all drugs, it should only be used for its proper purpose. This is to help men who suffer from physically related impotence, not to let 70-year-olds imagine they are 17.

Viagra has side-effects that can include distortion of colour vision and headaches. One of the main drawbacks concerns men with heart and circulation disorders. Such people may well be among those longing to take the drug because they have experienced impotence either as a result of poor circulation or from treatment for hypertension. Unfortunately, Viagra causes a sudden fall in blood pressure and for men who have these medical conditions the results could prove fatal.

At the time of writing, Viagra has been associated with some 140 deaths worldwide. Viagra, in fact, should not be taken in conjunction with any other nitrate or nitrite product, such as 'poppers', or other drugs which lower the blood pressure. Although Viagra will do nothing to help improve communications skills and somewhat over-stresses the male sexual performance, both parties in a relationship may be grateful that the man has been aided to rediscover his powers by this product.

QUESTION 6

Can a young woman ever truly fancy an older man?

Certainly there is no law specifying an age barrier or 'sell-by' date for love. Theoretically, anyone can fall for anyone. A cynic would say it helps if the older man is rich and successful. Money and power have long proved aphrodisiacs. Young women seeking emotional and material security would naturally respond to partners who can provide both. It's perfectly natural for girls who have had only brief contact with their fathers, or whose families have broken up, to seek for fatherly qualities in some of their partners. An optimist would point out that older people can impart wisdom and joy of experience to younger lovers.

Older women in their sexual prime at 40 can take younger men, in their prime at 20, to the outer limits of erotic pleasure. Older men – able to last longer – can transmit these secrets to young girls, who may possibly benefit from a gentler introduction to the arts of love.

QUESTION 7

What if I don't fancy my partner any more?

Don't be too hasty to rush to conclusions. The urge to fancy somebody is composed of many different feelings, some of them hard to influence, but several of them much easier to change. If you have had a recent emotional disturbance like a bereavement, or have lost your job, it is highly likely that you will have gone off sex, especially at home. The same applies if you're depressed. Some of the symptoms of depression may be hidden and require expert diagnosis and treatment by the doctor. If you feel resentful about your partner's recent behaviour or failure to appreciate you fully, this can also suffice to turn you off sexually.

As a general rule, sexual response is controlled by the wider emotions between the partners. But once you stop having sex – perhaps because you are bored with the sexual routine – the *not* having sex can become a problem by itself. It then takes a conscious decision to go to bed and 'restore the habit' to overcome the problem. Don't forget, there's nothing wrong with asking your partner to help by dressing to please or in varying the sexual routine. If you attempt to make love in the same way every single time, you *will* grow tired of it.

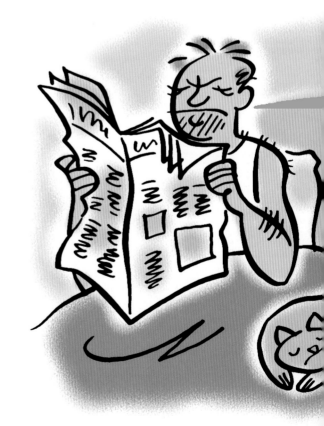

Why doesn't my partner fancy **ME** any more?

Be sure you're decoding the signals accurately. When women go off sex it's often because they're unhappy with the general state of their relationship. You cannot shout and scream at her one minute and expect loving submission the next. Cast your mind back over the past few days. How much friction has there been? Put this right if you can. Don't forget that grudges can be harboured for months. Work on respect. Try to think of your lover as a stranger you'd like to impress rather than a companion it's easy to take for granted.

Other things to consider – do you make love to her in the way that she likes? Can you be sure? If in doubt, play the game one night of letting her direct you (like air-traffic control) to pleasure her body. Call this by some romantic name (like 'the secret garden') and you''ll probably re-kindle lost interest. Demonstrate your love and you'll almost certainly get more sex. Remember, all desire fluctuates, but most people respond to a mix of massage, attention, honesty and humour.

If none of this works, it could be time for a serious heart-to-heart and/or counselling to find out what is really going on in your relationship.

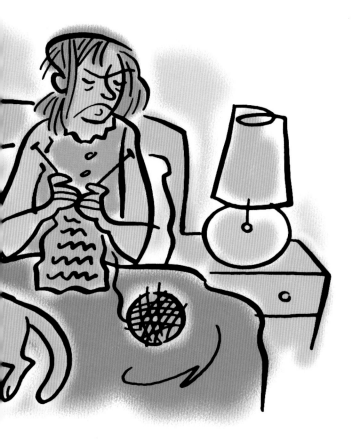

If neither my partner nor I want sex any more does it really matter?

No, because the bad stress of doing something neither of you wants would outweigh the emotional and physical benefit of regular intercourse. Making love *on demand* is a perversion. If gardening gives you more pleasure, then gardening it shall be. Were there any truth in the rumour that celibacy is a health risk, we'd find monasteries full of the lame, the sick and the prematurely deceased, which we don't.

However please be sure you have really given up, with no desire even for masturbation. Some people 'go off sex' out of excessive self-consciousness or embarrassment. These are problems that should be taken to a therapist. The only trouble with *not* having sex in a long-term relationship is that you need to offer extra verbal and emotional reassurance. Sex is a kind of shorthand for showing your approval, and without it you need to compensate in so many other ways.

How can I keep going for longer?

Well, you could take Viagra, but nature has an easier way of helping if you obey your body's rules. It's important to understand that premature climax is partly an anxiety state. There's only one system of arousal in the human body and if a man is already worried about his sexual performance he is already half turned-on. When you start making love, you're probably closer to orgasm than you suspect.

So instead of leaping on your partner, you'd be better advised to lie gently with eyes closed, stroking each other's backs, synchronizing your breathing to hers and helping your system to restore a little bit of order. Then practise the 'stop-start' method of control. As you feel yourself reaching the 'point of no return', when ejaculation is inevitable, cease moving altogether and let the erotic sensations subside. When you feel the tension ease, gently resume rocking or thrusting. Quite by chance, this is likely to drive your partner to ecstasy, so has quite a lot to recommend it. Teasing is at the heart of erotic love. Men with premature ejaculation are advised to give their partners masses of pleasure – and orgasm – before penetration.

LONG-TERM RELATIONSHIPS

OVER HALF OF ALL MEN IN MID-LIFE ARE WITHIN A LONG-TERM RELATIONSHIP, HAVING BEEN WITH THE SAME PERSON FOR TWO, THREE, EVEN FOUR DECADES. AS WE'VE SEEN, MEN WITHIN SUCH A RELATIONSHIP TEND TO LIVE LONGER – BUT DO THEY FEEL YOUNGER? WE LOOK AT KEEPING THE FUN AND THE NOVELTY IN LONG-TERM LOVE.

BEATING BOREDOM

Scratch the surface of many a contented long-term partnership and you will find a man who feels bored and prematurely 'middle-aged' – while having no real desire to split from his 'other half' and a great deal of affection for that partner still. Why *do* long-term relationships often make you feel stale and bored? And what can be done about it?

The fact is that we spend more time servicing our cars than our personal partnerships, and any relationship will grow stale if it is neglected. Sometimes we need to re-invest rather than taking each other for granted. In other words, it is relationships that need 'tender loving care' as well as individuals.

One good idea is to sit down together and make positive decisions about breaking the cycle of neglect. Plan your goals for the next six months. Review the way you treat each other. Topics to consider and talk through are:

● The balance of work and play. If you are working too hard or too long the boredom could stem from that rather than simply your relationship. Couples who do enjoyable things together enjoy each other more! Ask yourselves what you most enjoy and do more of it – dancing, sailing, bridge, playing the stock market – whatever. Focus on what works.

● Creating time off from parents and children. How long since you were properly alone together to talk, reminisce, have fun, relax, be yourselves? If you still care enough to want to stay together, there must still be some basic attraction. Plan to take regular time off together and re-awaken that attraction.

● Creating time off from each other – if you are with each other all the time, that can create the illusion of staleness. No individual can possibly supply all your needs in this life, and every couple needs to take some time off from togetherness to appreciate the finer points of each other and of home. Plan for each of you to have time to do something by yourselves, or with other people, at least a once a week.

● Investing time and effort in listening to your partner's daily concerns – how well do you really know what is going on in your partner's mind? How long since you talked about anything apart from the mundane things of everyday life? See 'We Don't Talk Any More' on the right.

● Reducing the number of negative remarks that you make to each other. Try not to moan and groan about life and/or each other all the time. Try to be positive, not negative and enthuse about the good things in your life rather than moaning about the bad – at least some of the time.

● Remembering to make small gestures of love and esteem. Think back to how you felt when you were 'courting' and what you did – the notes, the little gifts, the phone calls, the nicknames, the hugs . . . do it again.

Failure in these areas gets in the way of even wonderful partnerships, and features in the early stages of separation and divorce. Get in the habit of putting aside a time every week for one-to-one discussion and planning.

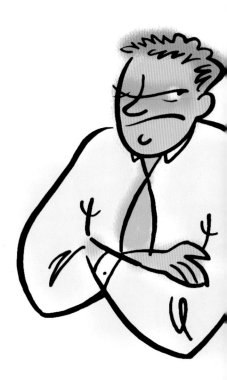

WE DON'T TALK ANY MORE

Some partners are silent in case they say too much. They fear personal conflict or were even brought up to think that nice people don't have rows. Men, in particular, like to avoid emotional confrontation at home because they get flooded with aggressive hormones that take a long time to dissipate, whereas women have far less testosterone to worry about.

It is also said that men 'lack the words and skill' to talk about their feelings. However, it doesn't take the brain of an Einstein to sit down and say something like, 'How are you? How do you feel about us? Are you and I a good pair? Do you still feel happy? What problems do you see ahead? Is there any-thing I could change about me to help solve them? Where do you see us heading as a couple? Do you like living with me? Can I tell you what is bothering me?' Practise asking at least one direct question like these on a regular basis and build on the answers – bearing in mind that, if you haven't talked in ages, your partner may take a while to realize that you really do want to know the answers. You do – don't you?

To Love or to Leave?

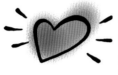

Perhaps you feel that your relationship has gone beyond just boredom – you are actually indifferent to one another, maybe you're in conflict, or you feel that you are just not getting on any more. Is it time to think about splitting up?

All relationships go through 'cycles of intimacy and distance' and there will be times when you two feel less than close. There will also be occasions when one or both of you feel(s) resentful because of underlying or unresolved conflicts. These may be sorted out if you can open or re-open the lines of communication between you. It doesn't matter what's happened – a lie, a betrayal of trust, money pressures, an affair, or just long-term taking your partner for granted – things can be put right so long as you are prepared to be honest with your partner and listen to their concerns.

This means *not* denying anyone's feelings, however uncomfortable or irrational they sound. When your partner says they feel upset, that is a fact. There's no point in replying 'But you don't need to be upset – I've changed.' People move on at different rates. What's water under the bridge for you may still be a flood alert to them. You cannot undo the past but you can help change someone's troubled feelings by giving them emotional respect.

If you can't sort out your problems together, following the guidelines opposite, one possible solution is for both of you to consult a therapist or counsellor. It would also be important to overhaul the *rest* of your life to make sure there is good stimulation – fun – as well as stress. And to bear in mind that we also need to grow up enough to recognize that some of our choices can't be unpicked so easily. If we have children, for example, they cannot be divorced and, for the time being, we need to consider putting up with some heartache for their sakes. If the relationship has really gone sour and you have to remain under one roof for the sake of economy or the children, try not to dump all the blame on your other half. Nobody ever got married in order to make their partner's life hell.

Lastly – everyone will make a mess of at least one relationship in their lifetime. In American business, it is important to have experience of being fired or you may not get hired. The same principle applies to relation-ships – if you haven't been round the block a few times before settling down, it's reasonable to expect a few additional problems.

THINGS TO ASK YOURSELF
BEFORE EMBARKING ON AN
EXTRA-MARITAL AFFAIR

● Are things still tolerable at home? Do you still have love and/or affection for your partner? How would you feel to see her upset or even made ill or suicidal by your affair? If you would feel sad or upset at causing her misery, it is worth reconsidering.

● How will you feel about continually lying to your partner? Guilt and constant lies can put a cloud over the most passionate of affairs. And, if and when your long-term partner finds out, many women say that it is having been lied to that damages the marriage much more than the physical act of sex with another person. So, unless you don't mind losing and/or hurting your partner, don't start the affair.

● Do you feel any doubts about your love for this new person? Be honest – is there even some element of trying to feel young again? If you feel panicky about growing older, remember that nothing dates a man like taking a young woman to bed to compete with younger rivals.

● Are you primarily tempted by sex? If it is new kinds of sex that tempt you, it's surprising how many wives and partners, when told about an affair, say, 'You know, I'd been dying to do that with you for years!' Still going ahead? If you still mean to go ahead, the only compensating thought is that many long-term relationships are bound to break up and others only survive by compromises – including infidelity.

Affairs – Can They Be the Answer?

Many a man will say 'yes'. In her book *Adultery*, Annette Lawson showed that although extra-marital affairs usually cause misery, this isn't enough to stop people having them. Nor do those involved express much regret. The pay-off appears to outweigh the pain.

So why do people do it? For most of us, life is an emotional struggle. We feel deprived of attention and terrified that 'this is all there is'. So occasionally, we press the panic button. We attempt to 'star in our own movie'. We turn on the heady adrenaline of falling in love. More importantly, we turn on the heavy adrenaline of having someone fall in love with *us*. We relax our rules on promiscuity at times when our identities are under threat – after divorce, during pregnancy, when we lose a job, when a parent dies, when we age, as life gets dull. This is the pattern – although we remain free to make individual choices.

An affair is basically a 'new beginning', reviving for a moment the early rapture of teenage passions. On this analysis, if adultery were more acceptable, it would be less popular!

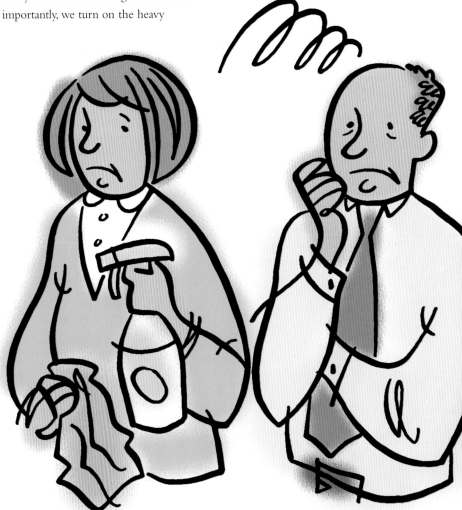

Best of Both Worlds

An affair is by no means always the result of a bad marriage. Many men in mid-life embark on an affair even though they still feel love and affection for their long-term partner. In such instances, can an affair ever be worth the likelihood of future misery for all concerned?

Certainly, an affair can never be 1,000 % 'safe'. However far from home you go and however unlikely your partner is to find out, there is always some risk of discovery. So if you are thinking of beginning an affair so that you can have your home comforts and your passion, hoping never to be discovered, think again. If you *are* discovered, you may be lucky and find that your long-term partner is forgiving – but you may not. Things will certainly never be quite the same in the marital home again.

Consider the amount of lying that will be required. To start with, lying isn't easy unless you're an expert. The story you concoct to cover your tracks has to be consistent forever. And when you sleep with someone, you also sleep with everyone they've ever slept with, and you could catch a disease.

The price of an affair is the maximum damage it is likely to cause. This can only be calculated on a 'worst case' basis. Double-check your motivation.

Perhaps instead of asking yourself 'Is an affair worth it?', you might ask 'Why am I considering having an affair?' – and then make some changes in your life so that you don't. This could even include divorce and a new lover, or it could be you need to change your home or your job. You could just need two weeks in Greece. At the very least, first ask yourself the questions in the panel on the left.

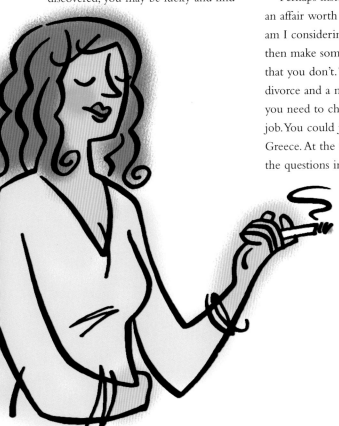

THINGS TO ASK YOURSELF BEFORE LEAVING THE MARITAL HOME

So you've decided that your marital problems can't be resolved – or you went ahead with the affair and got found out, or you fell so much in love that you can't see any other answer than to leave home. Here are a few last-ditch things to consider.

When you abandon a marriage, you tend to lose more than you may realize at the time. A very high percentage of divorced men say they regret breaking up. They wished they could turn back the clock. By opting for a clean break, it may appear that you are solving problems to do with conflict and bad sex. However, you are also cutting ties with home, family and the very social network that supplies your identity.

Are you ready for such a huge change, with its almost inevitable backwash of bereavement and depression? This *is* a step of last resort. Ask yourself if you could be feeling low for other reasons which a separation will not cure. What makes you believe the grass is going to be greener when you finally get together with your new companion?

Ask yourself these questions about her and your new relationship:
- Have you seen her under conditions of stress?
- Have you shared her daily routine?
- What is she like when ill?
- How bad a temper does she have?
- Has she any gift for compromise?
- Will she enjoy and respect your children?
- Will she say sorry when in the wrong?

These simple components of everyday life actually make the difference between joy and misery. It would be unwise to step from the frying pan into the fire.

WEIGHING UP THE YOUTH FACTOR IN YOUR RELATIONSHIP

Ring the answer nearest the truth for each of the 10 questions below, add up your score and then check your Youth Factor opposite.

1. *Do you throw a surprise party for your partner:*
- ☐ Often?   *score 2*
- ☐ Sometimes?   *score 1*
- ☐ Never?   *score 0*

2. *Do you plan an evening or day out for you and your partner (choosing and organizing it all yourself):*
- ☐ Often?   *score 2*
- ☐ Sometimes?   *score 1*
- ☐ Never?   *score 0*

3. *Do you buy new clothes from fashionable shops:*
- ☐ Often?   *score 2*
- ☐ Sometimes?   *score 1*
- ☐ Never?   *score 0*

4. *Do you change your hairstyle:*
- ☐ Often?   *score 2*
- ☐ Sometimes?   *score 1*
- ☐ Never?   *score 0*

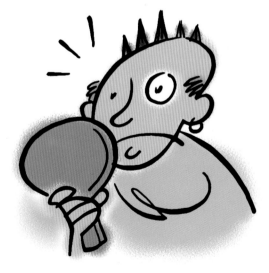

5. *Do you make love at times other than night-time:*
- ☐ Often?   *score 2*
- ☐ Sometimes?   *score 1*
- ☐ Never?   *score 0*

6. *Do you ask for what you enjoy when having sex:*
- ☐ Often?   *score 2*
- ☐ Sometimes?   *score 1*
- ☐ Never?   *score 0*

7. *Do you feel pangs of jealousy when your partner flirts with someone else:*
- ☐ Often?   *score 2*
- ☐ Sometimes?   *score 1*
- ☐ Never?   *score 0*

8. *Do you buy romantic music for your partner:*

☐ Often?   *score 2*

☐ Sometimes?   *score 1*

☐ Never?   *score 0*

9. *When you've been apart for a while, do you look forward*
to seeing your partner again:

☐ Often?   *score 2*

☐ Sometimes?   *score 1*

☐ Never?   *score 0*

10. *Do you say or write loving/romantic things to your partner:*

☐ Often?   *score 2*

☐ Sometimes?   *score 1*

☐ Never?   *score 0*

YOUR SCORE   ☐

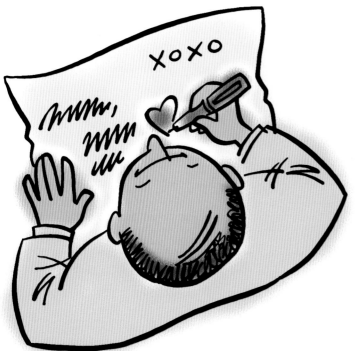

Your Relationship's Youth Factor

If you scored
between 15 and 20:

Your relationship is by no means making you feel old before your time! You seem to invest as much thought and passion into your partnership now as you did when you first met. Your enthusiasm is no doubt rewarded with a delighted and youthful partner, too, and a fun and happy marriage that should last as long as you do – which will no doubt be a few decades yet!

If you scored
between 8 and 14:

Like most of us, there are times when you feel that your relationship is getting a bit stale and that it needs livening up. The fact is that most of the answers are in your own hands. You're still young-at-heart some of the time – but don't feel you have to 'act your age'. You can still have fun and endless pleasure with your partner if you think you can.

If you scored
under 8:

Have you given up on life, or just on your relationship? However fit and healthy you are – your Real Age is old! At the very best, you are taking your partner for granted and taking life far too seriously. At worst, you are in grave danger of having her run off with the milkman or a colleague – whoever shows her a bit of fun and affection. Loosen up a bit – relationships only atrophy if you let them.

STARTING OVER

SO YOU'RE OUT OF THAT RELATIONSHIP AND 'STARTING OVER'. THOUGH MOST MEN LEAVE ONE PARTNER TO GO WITH ANOTHER, THERE ARE ALSO LOTS OF MEN WHO FIND THEMSELVES ON THEIR OWN AT THE END OF A LONG-TERM PARTNERSHIP – OR ELSE THE NEW LOVE AFFAIR HAS ALREADY GONE WRONG, AND THERE YOU ARE, BACK FACING THE DATING GAME. HERE'S OUR GUIDE TO GETTING IT RIGHT.

Forgive yourself for feeling like a duck out of water. It's a long time since you had to fend for yourself. You're not very used to feeling like a novice, so this will, of course, add to the anxiety. However, these concerns disappear as soon as you successfully circulate, and before long you will wonder what your worry was.

Over the last 20 years or so, dating has changed in response to society. The family has changed shape in that time and rates of divorce are still high, especially for the 30–40 age group. One consequence for men is that there are lots of 'spare' individuals from which to choose.

Start by getting in touch with any other friends who have travelled the same route. Go out with mates who can show you the ropes. Rehearse a few phrases for when you do get in touch with possible new partners:

● *'I'm newly separated and I feel a bit rusty'.*
● *'Please don't think me strange, but I'm a little shy.'*

If your lifestyle doesn't seem to present you with many suitable opportunities for meeting new people, it is perfectly acceptable to use a dating agency (make sure it is properly registered and with plenty of people for you to meet in your own area) or you could even ask your computer to find you a companion.

THE DATING GAME

There are very few rules in the 1990s on dating – certainly few rules of romantic etiquette. Being honest (being 'yourself') works best because you get what you want rather than playing games. As for sex and love, most people need to know where they stand. If you simply want sex, that's cool. People can say yes or no. If you really want to get married, that's cool too. But implying you want marriage in order to get sex – that isn't cool.

Anyone can date anyone, gay or straight. Age gaps no longer make a difference. Couples can share a hotel bed for the weekend without making love while others have sex on the first date. There's less pressure in so many ways that we all ought to feel more free

Two rules do remain: you cannot refuse to wear a condom if you expect to have sex – it's not negotiable; and women do not like being jumped on after a first, second or third date, unless they initiate the contact.

The science of attraction

If you believe the research on heterosexual love and attraction, the secret is a combination of financial solvency, a sense of humour and an attractive bottom. Men constantly worry that women need to be impressed by their virility, but what women actually say they want is a man who is romantic rather than raunchy. Women remain unimpressed by male genital proportions, except as an occasional talking point!

Facial beauty doesn't even come into it, so forget plastic surgery. If you are going to spend money on your desirability, take a course in psychology or counselling. One important fact is that women seem to prefer men who show their vulnerabilities – which is basically why they sometimes choose a weak rotter over a stuffed shirt.

However, there is one flawed assumption behind this question. No individual male will *ever* be desirable to *all* women. Tastes vary too much. So don't be depressed if you sometimes get rejected. Your ideal partner is going to have a personality very similar to yours – with the same preferences in most areas, from religion to food – but that leaves a lot of people with whom you cannot and won't get along.

And what turns people off ...

Women's biggest complaints about men include 'lack of respect' and 'lack of intimacy'. Nobody, in effect, likes to be taken for granted or ignored. The great psychologist Alfred Adler once said that what makes the world go round is attention – and we all need more of it.

Men who broadcast their egos non-stop

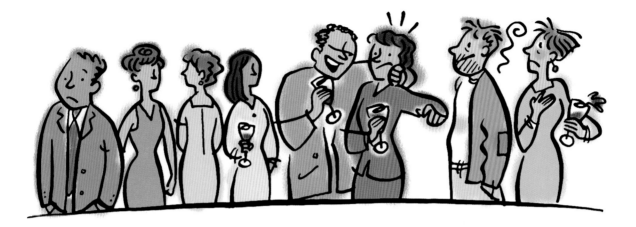

obviously run into trouble. However, many men also say things like 'I'm only working 18 hours a day for you and the kids, you know!' when what they really mean is 'I enjoy being a workaholic – at your expense.'

Gender differences affect the sex battle. Put crudely – men need sex in order to express their feelings and women tend to prefer emotional contact before they feel like having sex. A wise man understands and accepts this.

Other trivial though important turn-offs are reported to be men who smell bad (not just BO but also stale tobacco, last night's alcohol or curry), men who don't keep themselves reasonably well groomed, (i.e. dirty hair, teeth, nails or clothes), men who don't keep themselves maintained (e.g. bad teeth, pot bellies).

Conversely, vain men are also a no-no! Don't let her catch you admiring yourself in the mirror too often or worrying about your hair getting mussed up when you make love!

Avoidance of hurt . . .

What you want to know when you embark on a new affair is how can you avoid getting hurt. Of course you do.

First, respect your emotions. There's little point in rushing into a new life of dating when you still feel battered by some recent break-up. Take time to mourn. See why things went wrong and admit your failings. If you don't learn from your mistakes you're likely to repeat them.

Second, when you do start seeing new friends and potential partners, tell them what you've been through rather than pretend to survive unaffected. This will save you from trying to deliver more than you can perform, especially in bed. It often feels awkward to make a fresh start, and odd to touch new bodies. So don't set the standards sky-high at the outset. 'Divorce impotence' is common enough without you joining the list of sufferers.

Ultimately, of course, there is no way of eliminating all risk of a broken heart. If you never open yourself up to romantic rejection you can never fall in love either – it goes with the territory. Just remember that human beings are resilient and so long as we pace ourselves properly we can survive most reverses.

Nothing's working . . .

If you have been 'starting over' for some time without much success at all in the romance or sex stakes, you may be wondering what you are doing wrong. It could be that you are doing nothing wrong. Walk into a room containing 100 people and the chances are that you could only have a successful and close relationship with about three or four of them. With the rest, you have too little in common.

On the other hand, it always feels bad to invite failure, and you'd obviously like to minimize the likelihood of rejection. The main mistake men make is trying too hard to impress a potential partner. You stop 'being yourself'. It may be fun for an evening, yet nobody really wants to go out long-term with a 'performer'. 'Who is this man?' they wonder. So the best advice is to stop thinking about *yourself* entirely.

Successful men know how to listen to others, take an interest in their lives and ask open-ended questions like, 'Tell me what's happening in your life'. They also have expressive, mobile faces that acknowledge what is being said to them. So if you really want to make people want you, don't focus on yourself.

self

who are you? where are you?

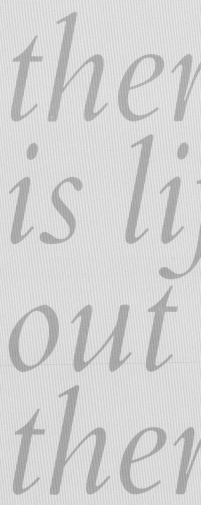

Who are you? Not the same person you were at 20 or 30, that is for certain. You have evolved into what you are today – but are you happy with that? Where are you? Has life turned out how you planned – and is it still what you want? Or did you not do any planning – and are now not sure where to begin?

The male menopause is now a recognized fact of life for very many men and can begin as young as 40 or occur much later. At some time during this period – and for some men this can span several years – you realise you are changing. Some see it positively, as maturing; others negatively, as decline.

There is much discussion about whether this reduction in drive and energy for many men is related to the depletion of testosterone, or whether the general ageing process – or, indeed, psychological factors – are the cause. In all probability it is a combination of all three. However – as many dynamic men in their 40s, 50s 60s and over have proved – there *is* a life out there if you want it.

Another symptom of the male menopause is a restless urge for chucking out the old (wife, job, home) and bringing in the new. This is an urge that can be positive if channelled properly – otherwise it can be very destructive indeed.

In other words, most men in their mid-life years find themselves considering goals, values, lifestyle; worrying about self-worth, achievements, the future . . . And that is what this section is all about – helping you to find balance, harmony and worth within your life, as well as interest, novelty, excitement and challenge, fun and relaxation. It's about self-reassessment, promoting the positive sides of your life, and learning how to cope with – or eliminate – the negatives which can result in stress and depression.

You can't turn back the years, but you can take stock and move on to where you want to be. My thanks to Phillip Hodson for his help with parts of the text.

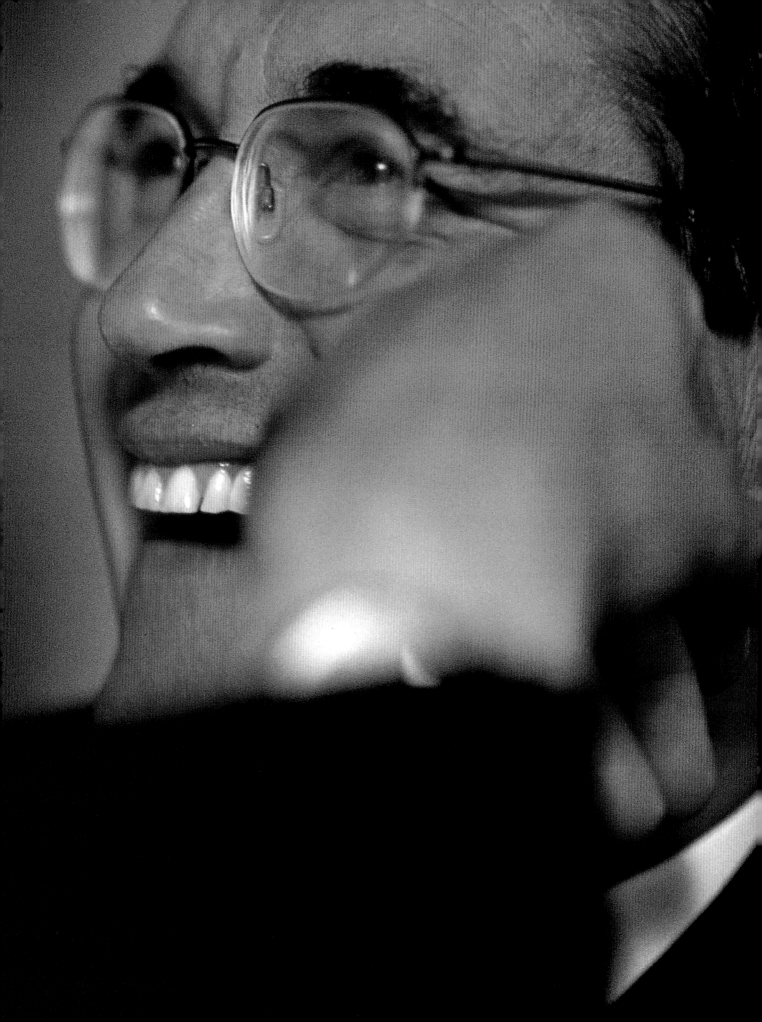

SELF-ASSESSMENT QUESTIONNAIRE

NOT EVERYONE HAS THE SAME SET OF WORRIES – USE THIS QUESTIONNAIRE TO ASSESS THE AREAS OF YOUR LIFE IN WHICH YOU PROBABLY NEED TO MAKE CHANGES. ANSWER THE 10 QUESTIONS HONESTLY AND THEN CHECK THE RESULTS TABLE TO SEE WHAT AREAS OF THE SELF SECTION WILL BE MOST RELEVANT TO YOU.

Tick your answers as you go.

1. Which of the following statements most matches your attitude to taking up a new hobby or interest?

☐ a   Too old; can't be bothered; nothing I fancy doing comes to mind.

☐ b   I'm always looking for new challenges.

☐ c   I haven't time for hobbies – I'm far too busy with work.

☐ d   I need to relax in my spare time, not take on even more stress!

2. Which of the following most describes your feelings on a work morning when you wake up?

☐ a   Keyed up, tense, worried.

☐ b   No thought at all about the day ahead, claustrophobia, boredom, resentment.

☐ c   Don't work (redundant, retired, etc.).

☐ d   Look forward to the day.

3. How would you describe your attitude towards your financial situation?

☐ a   Worry about money – or lack of it – all the time.

☐ b   Careful about saving up every spare penny for the future.

☐ c   I'm quite happy but I am fairly careful with what I have.

☐ d   I often overspend/get in debt, but it doesn't bother me.

4. At work, which description best matches how you think others see you?

☐ a   Self-confident, able, respected.

☐ b   Invisible, taken for granted.

☐ c   Willing, trusted, liked.

☐ d   Don't work.

5. After work, which of the following are you most likely to do?

☐ a   Go for a drink near work with colleagues.

☐ b   Go home/watch TV/fall asleep.

☐ c   Go home then later go out somewhere with friends/partner.

☐ d   A regular mix of all of these.

6. How many days off work have you had in the past year, other than legitimate holidays or acute/real illness (e.g. flu, broken leg)?

☐ a   More than 10.

☐ b   About 2 or 3.

☐ c   None.

☐ d   Don't work.

7. If your close family had to describe you, which do you think they would say most closely matches your behaviour/attitude at home?

☐ a   Bossy, distant, organized, selfish.

☐ b   Kind, fun, hands-on, generous.

☐ c   One of the kids, disorganized, extravagant.

☐ d   Don't have close family.

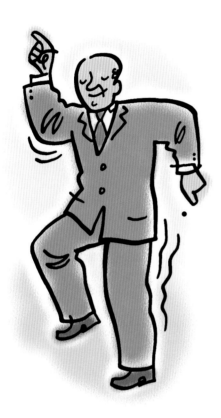

8. *After a hectic week with no time to spare on yourself, you suddenly have a few free hours. Which of the following would you be most likely to do?*

- a Watch TV, do nothing, sleep.
- b Read, listen to music, phone friends.
- c Drink alone.
- d Go out partying.

9. *If a particularly busy day at work crops up, which of the following are you most likely to do to get through the workload?*

- a Recruit extra help/delegate.
- b Get in early and leave late, when it is all done.
- c Cancel lunch-date with old friend and miss your gym class to give yourself extra time.
- d Nothing – do what you can and leave what isn't done to pile up, even though it may make matters worse next day.

10. *Which of the following best describes your sleep patterns?*

- a Can't get off to sleep easily, and/or wake up in middle of night and can't get back to sleep.
- b Sleep fine most nights without the aid of sleeping pills.
- c Sleep okay, but don't like waking up/getting up in the morning.
- d Sleep with the aid of pills.

RESULTS

Circle the number given for each of your answers.

statement	a	b	c	d
1	1	0	4	2
2	4	4	3	0
3	3	3	0	3
4	0	4	4	2
5	3	3	0	0
6	1,4	0	4	3
7	3	0	3	1
8	0	0	1	2
9	0	4	2	4
10	2	0	2	1,2

NOW Jot down how many 1's, 2's, 3's and 4's that you have circled.

- You can only circle one answer for each question.
- There is no need to add up the 0s.
- *If you have circled answer 6a, count that as one 1 and one 4 score.*
- *If you have circled answer 10d, count that as one 1 and one 2 score.*
- *The maximum number of 1's or 2's or 3's or 4's that you can score is 5.*

Number of 1's ☐   Number of 3's ☐

Number of 2's ☐   Number of 4's ☐

WHAT YOUR SCORE MEANS

If you scored any number 1's . . . .

You need to work on your lifestyle and personal problems – turn to Self-indulgence on pages 130–131. The pages on Relaxation (124–9) will also help you. If you scored 4 or 5 number 1s, give work on your lifestyle and personal problems a priority rating.

If you scored any number 2's . . . .

You need to work on your stress levels. Turn to Relax and Re-energize on pages 124–9 first and also read through the rest of this section to get tips on beating stress at work and at home. The piece on Self-indulgence (pages 130–131) will also help you to relax. If you scored 4 or 5 number 2s, pay attention to your stress levels as a priority.

If you scored any number 3's . . . .

You seem to be having trouble at home and/or with your finances. Turn to page 119 for advice on improving matters. The pages on Relaxation may also help you (124–9). If you scored 4 or 5 numbers 3's, sort out your home/money problems as a matter of priority.

If you scored any number 4's . . . .

You have work-related problems which should be addressed. Turn to pages 112–18 for help in the workplace. The pages on Relaxation and Self-indulgence will also help you (124–31). If work is making you hard to live with at home, also read pages 120–23. If you scored 4 or 5 number 4's, make it a top priority to sort out your work/career problems.

MEN AT WORK

WORK KEEPS MEN YOUNG BECAUSE IT SUPPLIES AN EMOTIONAL IDENTITY. WITHOUT AN IDENTITY YOU GET DEPRESSED AND FEEL USELESS. WORK CAN ALSO PROVIDE 'POSITIVE STRESS', STIMULATING THE BRAIN TO STAY ACTIVE AND YOUTHFUL. HOWEVER, WORK CAN ALSO BE THE CAUSE OF A GREAT DEAL OF NEGATIVE STRESS AND EMOTION, AND, IF IT'S ALL GOING WRONG, CAN ACTUALLY ADD TO THE FEELING OF 'GETTING OLDER'. HERE'S HOW TO MAKE WORK WORK FOR YOU.

WORK NEGATIVES AND HOW TO BEAT THEM

Boredom

Much of male mid-life crisis is to do with boredom, because you've been at the same old tasks for too long, or you haven't enough to do. If the thought of yet another day at work fills you not with anticipation or nervous energy, but enervating nothingness or the urge to rob a bank and escape to a life of adventure, then something needs to be done.

If one of the main problems is that you have to keep doing similar things – whether on a daily basis, a weekly cycle, or even if the same tasks come around with frightening regularity on an annual basis – see if you can organize new ways of doing the same old tasks. Whether it's new software, a new filing system, different order of work, or new ways of finding solutions – see what you can put in to make the job different and the work done better, and each task more satisfying for you.

Also, make quite sure that others know you are keen to do all this and that you are able to do it. Check out your visibility rating – are you one of the taken-for-granted, invisible tribe? Take a deep breath and test your voice, get opinions heard, make suggestions. Start

sending memos, suggesting meetings – get involved with what is going on again. *Ask* for more work.

Have you had promotion, or increase in salary, or a change in tasks within the last two or three years? If the answer is 'no', start asking yourself, 'Why not?' Whatever your age there is no real reason why you can't have one, two, or all of those things, except your own inhibitions and perhaps others' prejudices. If you're bored and it's your own business you're running, could you sell it? Could you do something new?

Make a game plan and go for what you want – as long as you believe it is feasible. In mid-life, particularly later mid-life, you *do* need to realize that the sky may no longer quite be the limit and your wildest ambitions may not quite be fulfilled. It is important to audit your activities and goals to suit what's possible.

Loss of ambition is nothing to be ashamed of, however. If you don't want the boss's chair or the move abroad, or whatever, it doesn't matter – as long as *you* don't mind. Along with the diminished testosterone levels, as already discussed, a down-sizing of your drive to reach the very top, and beyond, is a fairly

natural thing. There is no harm in reworking your plans regularly to fall just within – or right on the top edge of – real possibility.

Should you stay or should you go? If boredom is deep, there's little room for change and no chance of fat salary increases or more joy, many men – at any

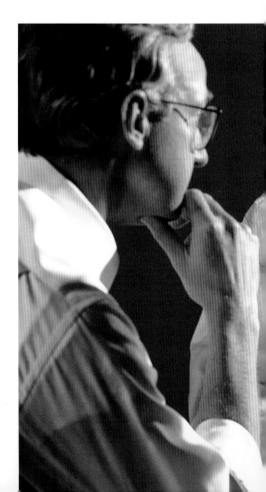

Resentment

age – feel like moving on.

Negative moves are to resign on the spur of the moment with nothing else in mind (don't do it!) and to antagonize everyone bearing in mind that you may want a good reference. Positive moves are to weigh up the pros and cons of leaving (write them down – but not on the company computer!) and then tackle the possibility of moving sensibly. Apply for new jobs. Go to interviews if you can get them, however unlikely it is that you may want that job – if you haven't moved workplace for years you need the practice. Don't resign until you've got something to go to (see also 'A Few Words About Self-employment' on page 116). Redundant, sacked? Use the tips in this section to help you cope.

You're bringing home the bacon and you're fed up with it. At 50 (say) you may have 30 years of constant work under your belt. Perhaps you have good reason to feel resentful and longing to do a Reggie Perrin.

The only course of action is to look at all the options (of which there are several) and decide what can be done in your own circumstances. Decide on the worst-case scenario if you follow any of the options and look at this both long-term as well as short-term.

❶ Have you enough money to retire or go part-time? This may necessitate a change in other circumstances (e.g. a move to a smaller home), but it may be more feasible than you think. For people who are truly work-sick, early retirement can be a great release, not 'the end of the story'.

❷ Would your partner – if you have one – like to take on more of the financial responsibility? As we head to the Millennium, it is no longer anything to be ashamed of if the female half of a couple is the main breadwinner. Forty per cent of women aged 35 and over are now chief earners in their households, and this is the most rapidly expanding group of the population. Just because a situation has always been the case in your household, it doesn't mean it can't change. Your partner may indeed relish the chance to take over the driving seat. Talk!

❸ Can you improve your job description so that you feel less resentment attached to it? Perhaps something less challenging (if you feel resentful and stressed out) or more challenging (if you feel resentful and bored, in which case follow the same thought processes as for Boredom (see left).

❹ How much do you value the lifestyle that your income generates? If the answer is 'a great deal', perhaps you may yet find a way to feel more comfortable and less resentful about continuing with your work. One man I know, when he feels hard done by takes a journey to see people living rough in the streets, or goes to a hospital cancer ward, or talks to people he knows who have been made redundant and would give their eye-teeth to be in work. Such visits give him the motivation to continue and make him realize he's being just a tad over the top in the self-pity department.

Lastly, spend plenty of time imagining yourself – in as much reality as possible – not in this current job. Maybe you'll feel useless. Maybe you'll feel depressed. Maybe you just need a decent, long break. Try the relaxation techniques on pages 124–9 and read the section on Self-indulgence (pages 130–131).

If you can think of hundreds of things you'd like to do were you not working so hard (or so often, anyway) and if most of those things are actually feasible (even when money is in shorter supply) – then you may well be ripe for a long-term change. See also the section on making the most of retirement and being out of work, 'Time to Kill', on page 123.

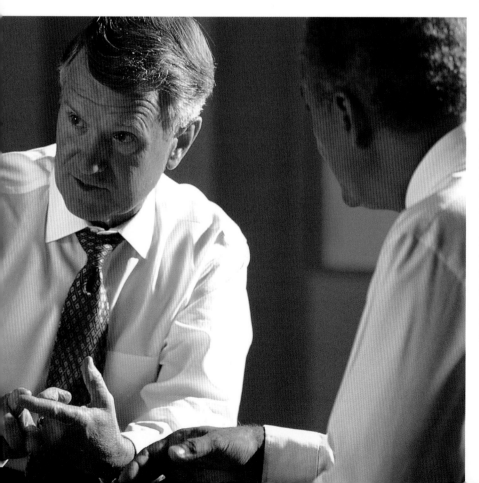

Keeping up with the competition

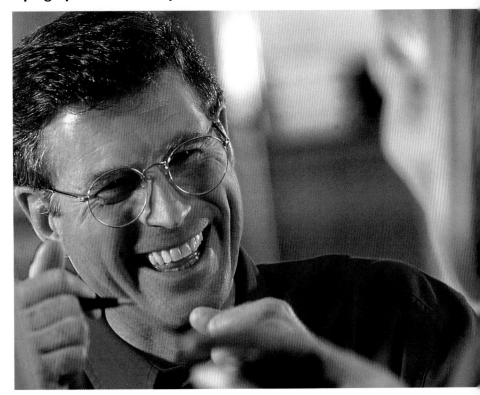

The stress of overwork is dealt with later in this section (on pages 116–7), but here we look at the stress of keeping ahead of the game when you are growing older and everyone around you seems to be growing younger.

The stress of such a situation can be even more acute if you work in a 'young person's' industry, such as the media or advertising, law or any physically demanding job. Then there is the thorny question of the recent explosion in jobs for women at all levels (if the statistics are to be believed), meaning that more and more men are having to learn to work along-side - or, indeed, for - females, when perhaps they had no need to do so until recently.

It is inevitable that the older you get, the more young people will be coming on behind you, and for most men (and, of course, women) that means people who want to show they are better than you, people who want *your* job. It is ironic that as you age, and the natural inclination for most men (with not enough raging hormones to spur you on) is to be slightly less competitive, you may feel as though you really need to be *more* competitive to stay on top.

Coping with ageing in the world of work is partly about pacing yourself and remembering the difference between quantity and quality – you have fewer physical units of energy available after 45, but you are just as intelligent as you ever were and probably have better judgement and more skill than youngsters (except in quick-reaction pursuits like maths, chess and bond-dealing).

Here are some practical points to consider and which may help:

● Write a list of all your good points at work, and why it is that you are the best at the job you do. This should help your self-confidence, lack of which is very debilitating at all levels of work. Keep reminding yourself of your assets all the time.

● If you think you are *not* the best, write another list of how you can improve your rating. This could be anything from seeking counselling for your lack of confidence to taking extra coaching in your poorer skill areas (with older people these are often areas involving new technology or practices). It is never too late to learn if you want to learn.

● Accept change in the workplace as

inevitable, useful and enriching. The person who hates change is likely to age quicker, and be less able to cope with incoming competition, than someone who looks upon it as a challenge.

● Look at your work performance as a knowledgeable outsider would look at it. What kind of report would you give yourself? Write up that report. If there is any room for improvement, go back to the previous item. Do the same report as if you were your boss (if you have one). You need to be open-minded and honest for this exercise to be worthwhile.

● If you are the boss of your own company (or self-employed) and have a nagging fear that competitors have the edge (perhaps your latest figures are telling

When your wife earns more than you do

Some men feel a shiver of fear (or, possibly, jealousy) when they find themselves in the position of having a wife or partner who is earning more than them and/or in a more senior position than them.

Advice? Relax and enjoy it! There are a lot of advantages to having such a partner, so think of the positives and build on those . . . better standard of living, less responsibility on you to provide, perhaps more time for *you* to do what you want, less tendency for your partner to be dependent, and so on. For some men, perhaps with a younger partner who is suddenly racing ahead while they feel things are slowly heading towards wind-up time, the situation may seem negative rather than positive. In that case you need to develop your sense of self as a whole person, not just as a work person. Alternatively, you may decide to use the female challenge to stir up your testosterone once more and take up that challenge, get the billions, the top job or whatever. It may be that you have been sitting on your laurels a bit after all?

You also perhaps need to do some work on why you feel so threatened by your partner's success. A marriage isn't a competition, it's a twosome.

And for any men who are finding it hard to work with, or alongside, colleagues who happen to be female – learn to live with it, it isn't going to change! Treat a woman like a colleague and she'll act like a colleague.

---

you so) you need to overcome the urge to bury your head in the sand, and do some espionage on other people's goods, prices, methods, perks, marketing – whatever. Don't be frightened to admit that you can improve. If you need help in taking on new challenges, read *Feel the Fear and Do it Anyway* by Susan Jeffries. At all costs avoid over-borrowing, overspending and over-drinking, and remember that redundancies and cutbacks are preferable to bankruptcy or re-mortgaging for the ninth time.

● If you are not performing well, is there a physical reason? Check out your fitness – a fit body really is an incredible asset in the workplace. If you look young for your age, too, that is a great help. The programme in this book should help to sort you out. Check out your diet (eat plenty of high-energy foods, such as whole-grains, fresh fruit and vegetables, pulses, nuts, seeds) and any niggling health worries.

If you feel tired all the time you won't perform well. Do you sleep all right (see page 127)?

If you are physically fit and sleeping well, yet feel tired, you need to break into the vicious circle of stress creating tiredness, in turn creating poor performance, which increases stress, which makes you feel more tired, which creates even poorer performance. Make regular time to relax and enjoy yourself and consider counselling if you are worrying all the time and feel stressed out.

A NEW JOB? WHAT YOU NEED TO KNOW

So you are looking for, or have found, that new job after years somewhere else (as our Case Study Roger describes overleaf). Here are a few pointers to success:

● Buy yourself some new clothes, get a haircut and get fit.

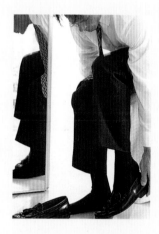

● Have a holiday.

● Bone up all you can on the company/job/ relevant skills if applying for a job, or before you start if you have been successful.

● Be persistent. Although new guidelines (in the UK) should make it easier for people of 45 and over to find a new job, ageism is still rife. Promote your energy as well as your experience and reliability.

● Once you have the job, keep a low profile for the first week or two. Case the joint. Sum up the people.

● Try not to panic if you feel like you did on your first day at big school. It will pass.

● Be sociable in a laid-back kind of way. Remember to treat women as colleagues – not potential girlfriends.

A few words about self-employment

Many men in mid-life, having worked for someone else for years, dream of going self-employed. It can work. Self-employment brings its own special benefits but also its own drawbacks, which you need to consider. If you are thinking of taking the plunge:

● Will you need an initial large outlay of cash to make the thing work? Have you got it to spare (or, worst-case scenario, to lose)?

● Will you need a great deal of energy and/or initiative to start it moving? If so, have you got that energy? Longer hours, at least at first, will be pretty inevitable.

● Can you cope with a lot of stress? Can you shoulder responsibility – and take the blame if things go wrong? Are you good at finding solutions to problems?

● If it does all go wrong, do you have a plan for what to do? Bear in mind that, if you are say in your 50s and giving up the 'regular job', it will be a lot harder for you to get another job later, than for someone in his 20s or 30s.

● Can you work well on your own, are you a self-motivator? Can you think for yourself without a boss/a meeting/etc?

Plus points of self-employment are the challenge, rekindling of interest in work (one hopes), working for yourself *can* be a great motivator for many people (although it can be extremely hard for others who have been used to working with colleagues for years), being your own boss is always extremely satisfying, and – hopefully – you will generate more money for yourself, if it all goes well.

Bear in mind that a very high percentage of new small businesses fail within two years of starting up. Feel the fear and do it anyway? Or make the most of what you've got? Take time before deciding.

Lastly a few words for the already self-employed. Your most likely problem is overwork and responsibility-related stress. Read on for ideas on dealing with both.

Overwork

A large proportion of working men – both bosses, staff and self-employed – complain about being overworked. It's probably the biggest gripe of all. But what exactly *is* overwork, in your view?

● Long hours?
● Few holidays?
● Few weekends off?
● Too much mental overload?
● Too much responsibility?

All of these together, or any of them in isolation, may feel like overwork to you. If you *feel* overworked you *are* over-worked, which will probably result in your having an unbalanced lifestyle, stress symptoms, and finally burn-out, exhaustion and depression.

It happens to a lot of men even as young as 35, successful or not so successful, rich or not so rich, high flyers or plodders. In the 20s and early 30s, natural energy, ambition and testosterone mean that you can keep up a phenomenal pace and take mega amounts of work-load and mental pressure. By the 40s for some and by the 50s and 60s for most, however, you realize that there really should be more to life than being dictated to by the need to earn money or the work ethic. That coupled with the natural decline in ambition for some, as already discussed, means that overwork can be badly tolerated and needs to be addressed if you are to enjoy life.

● Self-inflicted overwork is very common – and what you need to address here is *why*? You may be a victim of this type of overwork if you say yes to the following:

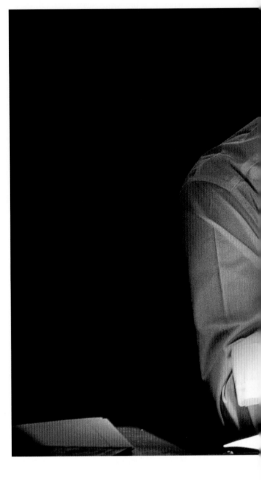

● You are the only one in your company who works so hard/so long.
● You are a perfectionist.
● You have trouble saying 'no'.

Many voluntary overworkers have a poor home or social life – they may be in a bad marriage (which, ironically, may be being made worse by the over-work itself), may be lonely, may feel socially inept.

Others may feel insecure in their own talents and need to do every job perfectly in order to justify their salary/position. Others may lack confidence to say no to long hours, overtime, taking work home at weekends, and so on. If you believe in yourself and your abilities, you won't fear the sack – or poor results

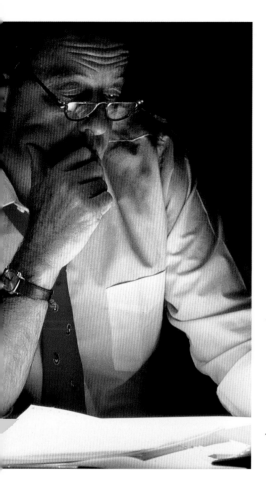

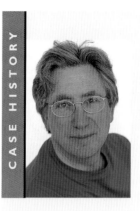

While building up a business, it is hard to take adequate time off. However, better time-management and stress-relief are both areas that should be explored (see the panel overleaf for time management and see pages 124–9 for Stress Relief).

● Slowing-down overwork is quite common in older people. This is when you take longer to do the same amount of work you used to do. Part of the reason for this could simply be boredom with the job – in which case turn back to page 112 for advice; otherwise, halt the natural decline in work-rate with a plan such as that in this book, overhauling all the following areas:

diet . . . a good wholesome diet, high in fresh fruit and veg and low in alcohol and junk, helps brain-power and energy levels.

amount of exercise you take . . . regular exercise, involving cardiovascular work (walking, cycling, etc.), will help energy, memory and concentration.

life outside work . . . a fulfilling, exciting life with plenty of new information input (e.g. through reading books, travel, meeting new people) helps maintain mental agility. Check out the ideas on page 123.

Relaxation . . . stress can hinder work-rate, as can poor sleeping patterns (probably stress-related anyway). Check out pages 124–9 for advice on relaxation.

sex life . . . good sex can help you work better. Check out pages 94–108.

● Outside influences can cause what may seem like genuine reasons to work long hours and never take holidays. For example, paying off debts, so that you have to take two jobs.

– if you stick to agreed hours. A good tip if you start a new job is to start as you mean to go on. Set achievable goals and don't allow yourself to accede to unreasonable requests.

Whatever the cause for your own self-inflicted overwork, it needs to be acknowledged and addressed. Don't moan – do something about it! Use the pointers above to decide just why you need to work so hard – then set about getting some balance back in your lifestyle (using this section to help you explore non-work facets of your life and character and to help you de-stress).

Bosses – whether self-employed or in charge of a huge company – are also often guilty of self-inflicted overwork.

Our participant Roger Douglas began his first full-time job for 16 years during our 10-week programme, at the age of 52. Having worked as a self-employed property consultant since his mid-thirties, during 1998 Roger decided that it really was 'time for a change'. After applying for some jobs on his own with no success, he joined the books of an employment consultancy and soon had a new job as a Building Project Manager in the public sector.

'I would advise anyone in a similar situation to find a job with the help of a consultancy rather than doing it alone. I feel that whatever your age, if you have clear objectives for the kind of job you want, and if you are qualified and perform well at the interview, then you can find work and it's never too late.

'One of the main reasons I wanted a change was that I felt like a new challenge, and I wanted more human contact; to be part of a team. Although the first few weeks were a sharp learning curve, I have all that now, and am loving almost every minute of it.'

TIPS FOR MANAGING YOUR TIME BETTER

● Plan ahead. Make lists and do the hardest tasks first thing in the day, when most people are at their best, freshest, most energetic and mentally alert.

● Decide how long tasks should take (whether written, oral, meetings, whatever) and stick to that.

● Delegate whenever possible.

● Be ruthless – don't waste time on people or involvements that aren't strictly part of your game plan (though bosses should always keep an ear to the ground for good business leads).

● Take short-cuts when you can. Sometimes less detail is better than more – learn to differentiate.

● Stay healthy in mind and body. A fit person manages time better than an unfit one.

So you are genuinely overworked. There is much you can do to ease the load. For one thing, remember that long hours and no vacations are a recipe for slowing down, anyway – and for making mistakes. Not taking time off may actually be a false economy of your own time. Regular short breaks during the day also help improve work-rate and quality.

For troubles with money – see opposite; much can be done to help here too.

For dealing with an unreasonable boss or unreasonable workload to which you seem unwittingly tied, try the following plan of action:

❶ State your case. Perhaps no one realizes how much work you are doing and how long it is taking you. State it first to the boss, in a calm but determined manner, and ask what he or she intends to do about it. Even better, state what you want to happen about it – e.g. more staff to help you cope; work shifted elsewhere. It always helps if you can think of solutions rather than forcing the boss to do some extra thinking.

Pointers for coping

❷ No joy? Take it higher (if there is a higher) or take it to your workplace representative, for example, a union or a personnel manager.

❸ If what may seem a normal workload to someone else is too much to you, consider job sharing, or seeing if there are any similar posts where you can work at a less frenetic pace.

❹ If there is a fine line between what is work and what isn't (e.g. you entertain clients a lot during the evening or at weekends, or you work abroad a lot) and there is no way round this, you need to press for longer holidays or periods of time off in return for working all hours when you need to.

❺ If you have been working somewhere for a long time and the lines are too thickly and indelibly drawn to be altered, you may have to consider moving.

Lastly, remember – the more successful you are, the *fewer* hours you should be working. Being overworked is not necessarily a sign of success or power. It could be a sign simply that you are just not being as clever as you could be!

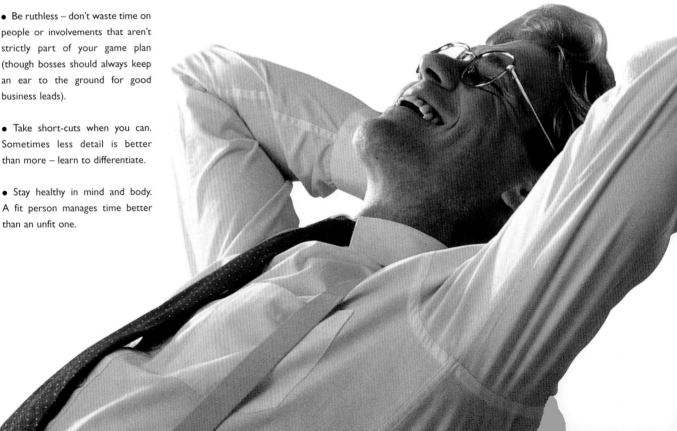

MONEY PROBLEMS

If you have money troubles they can invade every area of your conscious life. Here are a few tips that may help you sort out your finances.

If, however hard you work, you never seem to have enough money, it may be time to look at how you manage the money you do have, rather than expending all your effort on trying to get more.

A typical example is the household where both partners work and yet income is swallowed up by cleaners, gardeners, nannies, therapies to overcome the stress of burn-out, and on smaller things like labour-saving meals and taxis -- all necessary because you are both so busy. If you're not content, either, it makes no sense to continue feeling hard-pressed to earn a high salary when you're spending most of it on supporting a lifestyle that you really don't enjoy all that much.

If you are a home owner, you could probably make a great deal of money almost instantly by moving to a smaller home and/or to a less expensive area. This doesn't necessarily mean it is less nice. Sell a large family house in a London commuter area and buy a similar one in gorgeous Herefordshire, for example, at a quarter the price, and you will make enough profit to give you a reasonable income for life. Smaller homes also cost less to maintain and less to run, so you could think of down-sizing. If you are in mid-life, with children gone away or soon to go, these are the first options to look at, especially if you are retiring or can begin working from home.

You may also benefit from taking some time to look at other money-eating areas of your life that can be overhauled. Most professional people waste a great deal on clothes (how many in your wardrobe are never or hardly ever worn; how many items did you really need?), on wine, and on eating out a lot. Going out is good – but, if you often end a meal thinking you could have had much better at home and that you didn't really enjoy it, why not save money that way?

If you are now saying to yourself, 'But I've pared everything down and still haven't enough', the Citizens Advice Bureau can offer help on how to get started sorting your problems out in practical ways. Even if you are in debt or have a stack of full credit cards, it is always better to face true cash-flow problems rather than hide them away until they will, inevitably, get even worse.

RULE ONE
Overhaul your lifestyle and rationalize your spending.
Save what you can on things you don't really need or enjoy so that you can spend without guilt on things you really do need or enjoy.

In mid-life many people find that they wake up in a panic one night worrying that they haven't taken out enough pensions, peps, or whatever to ensure a comfortable life in retirement. If your money worries are centred on not having enough for the future, the obvious first step is to take financial advice and begin saving straight away.

However, the fear of not having enough money is nearly always worse than the reality. You may not need as much money as you think. Health insurance is the main consideration. Apart from that, the importance or other-wise of having large amounts of cash is largely related to your expectations.

A good exercise is to try altering your mind-set. How many instances can you think of where a low-cost alternative appeals to you as much as a high-cost option which also appeals to you. e.g. if you can't afford a holiday in Paris staying at the Ritz, a caravan touring holiday around the Dordogne might be even better; or if you can't afford to take a cruise round the Caribbean, you may see even more of interest (and get healthier) on a walking tour of Spain, or even your own locality.

As discussed above, your home is your greatest asset – if you own a property and want to enjoy life as you get older, sell it and think small.

A last thought about money in older age – freed from the every-day workplace, many third-age people find new talents and new ways to make money and find they enjoy their third-age careers or money-spinning hobbies more than they ever enjoyed their pro-fession. More on that on page 123.

RULE TWO
Save by all means, but don't think you can't have any fun if you aren't rich.
Which brings me on to the last consideration – that. however much you have, you can always find something to spend (waste) it on if you have a mind to. A few years back I saw a small piece of furniture in Harrods window as I walked by, with a £50,000 price tag. My first reaction was to feel inadequate. I imagined all these people wandering round Knightsbridge with enough money in their purses to buy a £50,000 piece of furniture with-out giving it a second thought. My second reaction was to realize that I didn't like the piece of furniture anyway, that I didn't want it or need it. My third reaction was to wonder at the stupidity of the consumer society, and I've never been near Harrods again. I guess the world *is* full of rich people looking for over-priced items to waste their money on.

As all research shows, however, richer people really aren't happier than the rest of us – but actually less cheerful and less content. My mother is one of the most contented people I know and takes a positive pride in living within her means (which are far from ample).

RULE THREE
Keep life simple. Real life is not material things, but the rest of it.
You know what I mean.

MEN AT HOME

AS FULL-TIME WORK FOR MEN AGED 40+ BECOMES MORE SCARCE (WITH, FOR EXAMPLE, 40% OF PEOPLE AGED BETWEEN 50 AND 64 IN THE UK NOT WORKING), MAN'S IDENTITY IS BECOMING MORE AND MORE LINKED WITH HIS ROLE AT HOME AND IN PERSONAL RELATIONSHIPS. WE LOOK AT THE CHANGING WORLD OF MEN AT HOME AND MEN WITHOUT WORK.

WAR OR PEACE?

Far from being the oasis of calm, comfort and harmony depicted in the TV ads, home life can be a great source of conflict and stress – and, therefore, ageing. Whether you are at home infrequently, or in frequent but short bursts, or there all the time, it is important to improve the quality of your home life and family relationships.

Are arguments necessary? Research by psychologist Dr John Gottman reveals that having *no* disagreements is a recipe for coma – in other words, the relationship probably has little depth.

He also says that 'silent avoidance' is one of the more damaging strategies for managing disputes. It's not the occurrence of the dispute that matters, but how you handle it. Handle disputes negatively (or pretend they don't exist) and matters will almost undoubtedly get worse; handle them positively and things should improve.

How many arguments begin:

- 'Why didn't you *tell* me? . . .'
- 'I didn't *know* that . . .'
- 'You *never* tell me *anything*!'

Disputes resolved by allowing each other to talk and explain, rather than loud negative accusatory shouting matches, are the goal to aim for. Whether the disagreement is about chores, kids, money, going out, habits, laziness, sex or work (these latter two dealt with elsewhere in the book) – or whatever – think 'talk'.

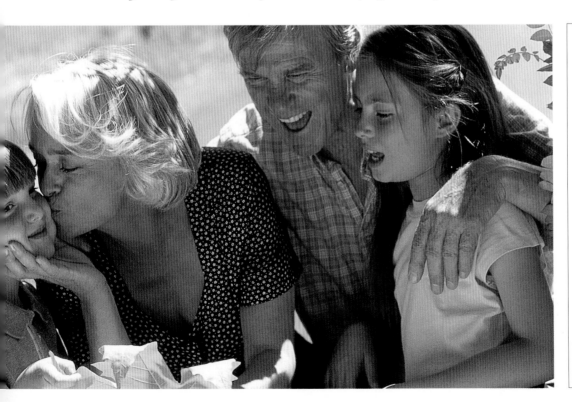

PLAYTIME

Every family needs to play together. If you only see each other in passing, or to row, or even to talk, you are missing out on one of the basic benefits of family life – people to do things with that are fun. Plan for regular time out together . . . outings, cinema, meals, walks, evenings at the pub – whatever. If you have time for fun and relaxation together it will reinforce the happy parts of your relationship. Whether you have just a partner, or children in their teens, or whatever, it is important to do this. And it's nice.

TALKTIME

Family talk-time is a good habit to get into – a regular 'slot' in your week, preferably when everyone is relaxed, that is set aside for discussion about any or all family matters. Think of it like a board meeting at home – when problems are aired, ideas and plans mentioned or put forward, possible causes for future disagreement ironed out, and so on.

Many families take each other for granted (compounded by separate, busy lives) and don't let each other know what is going on in their lives, either in the practical (real) sense or in their emotions. Talk-time was invented in the US to overcome this.

Talk-time is a very good occasion to sort out ground rules, especially in a new relationship but also in a long-term one. It is amazing how many long-term couples harbour resentment about all kinds of everyday chores like washing up, feeding the cat, picking dirty clothes up off the floor, etc., etc.

This is also a good time to discuss causes of resentment in families, such as one of you bringing unexpected guests back; differing ideas on what a good time to put the light out in the bedroom at night may be; how often or otherwise you both go out without the other; who decides what TV programme to watch, and so on. Deciding between you what is acceptable and what isn't when you are relaxed and on official talk-time is usually a good way to prevent many a row.

Talk-time only works if you are prepared to say what is on your mind. That goes without saying!

If you're thinking of doing something which you don't feel you can 'air' at talk-time – beware. It may be something you ought not to be thinking about doing, if your family happiness concerns you. Secrets lead to lies, lies lead to trouble.

Tips for solving disputes amicably:

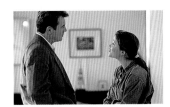

● Talk in a normal relaxed tone of voice and allow each other time to have your say.

● Listen to what the other person is saying.

● Try to look pleasant and receptive.

● Try to think of positive reasons why you disagree with what they are saying or asking for, if you do. For example, 'No you can't borrow my BMW to go out for the night because you are going to be drinking.'

● Try to offer compromise and/or alternative solutions. 'I'll order you a cab.'

● Try to find the hidden agenda. Many complaints that seem trivial or illogical are not really about the current problem but about wider or more long-standing problems.

● If there seems no solution at the present, terminate the discussion with, 'I don't think this discussion is getting anywhere at the moment – can we talk when we're not so tired/have more time/more chance to think things through'

● Book a time to have another go at finding solutions.

● Even better – have a regular weekly (or even nightly) 'talk-time' (see left), which should ensure that small disputes or problems don't turn into huge, unmanageable ones.

Of course, there may be problems that no amount of discussion can solve completely. If one of you admits to having an affair, or your partner wants her in-laws to come and live with you and you don't, for example, it may be that there is no easy solution. It may then be time to seek counselling.

CASE HISTORY

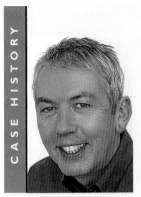

Noel Ahearne has been married to Lynne, 51, for 34 years, disproving the theory that young marriages rarely last. They have two daughters in their 30s, both married. 'Of course, every couple have their ups and downs but I think people give up too easily. What are our secrets for a happy home life? Well – I'm very easy-going (probably too much so!) and hard to argue with. I let it all wash over me and keep smiling.

'I've always tried to help around the home because I don't think it's fair that the woman should do it all. I actually like ironing – as long as I can watch TV while I'm doing it. I also enjoy cooking and when the girls were little I would change nappies and all that stuff. I came from a family of six children and there always seemed to be a baby around, so I learnt well then. I'm a bit untidy, Lynne says, but I do try to clean up after myself.

'I also think it helps to keep you together and happy if you have a good social life, which we do – a group of 16 friends have been meeting every Friday night for years – and we see a lot of the girls, and their husbands.'

10 personality traits worth developing
.... if you want to live happily within a family.

'Do as you would be done by' is an old but true homily. Hopefully, the other members of the family will reciprocate and be equally good to you.

❶ Thoughtfulness. People who don't bother with partners' birthdays, anniversaries, and so on, are not macho – just plain downright thoughtless. Also consider how you behave when your partner is ill, or worried, etc. Also think about other people's expectations as well as your own. If you are 'too busy' to be thoughtful with your loved ones, you aren't leading a balanced life.

❷ Willingness to compromise. You can't live within a group or a partnership without compromise or acquiescence. If all around you at home quake in their boots and bow to your every whim, stop feeling pleased with yourself – start compromising. If you want to be selfish, live on your own. If it is you who is doing all the compromising – start standing up for yourself.

❸ Willingness to share. Yes it is annoying if your son borrows your *Top Gear* magazine or your wife pinches your best sweater, but picture yourself living alone with your possessions all in perfect order. Might life be a trifle empty?

❹ Fairness. Try not to be unfair. If you make decisions others don't like, explain your reasons. If you haven't got a good reason, are you being fair?

❺ Calmness. It's not wonderful to live with someone who blows their top every few minutes over tiny things. Practise relaxation techniques or do whatever you must to help produce 'good vibes' in the house.

❻ Helpfulness. Not quite the same as thoughtfulness, helpfulness is perhaps more on the practical side of things. If you're both working, do you do a fair share of the chores or do you still expect your partner to do all the cooking, cleaning, family organizing, etc.?

❼ Kindness. Sometimes it is nice to be kind. It isn't true what you may have heard about women loving a brute! Most, in my experience (especially as they get older), prefer kindness above everything else.

❽ Sense of humour. If you can make the family laugh, they will forgive you a lot. Hopefully they don't need to. If the family can see *you* laughing, they'll be happy too . . . or, at least, happier than they would have been otherwise.

❾ Generosity. A mean man is a mean man is a mean man. Nobody likes meanness.

❿ Forgiveness. People in families make mistakes big and small. A bit of forgiveness for genuine mistakes and one-off moments of madness shows a true maturity. You care for your family 'warts and all' – just as they do you.

LIVING ALONE

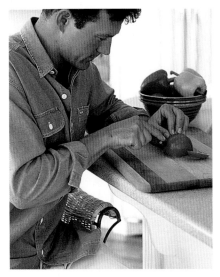

A fairly large percentage of mid-life men live alone. You are more likely to be happy on your own if this is by choice than if it is by accident. As we've already seen, married men are, on average, happier and live longer than single men.

If on your own, try recreating the family elements that are missing from your life – by encouraging a close circle of friends, by having them round to your home regularly, by going out together and by getting in the habit of regular intimate chat and swapping of problems. Also don't forget to follow the 'ten commandments' (left) with them – treat them well. Friends, relatives, grown-up children – all can be a rewarding family circle. If you do it right you can have the best of both worlds – a large and happy family and the relief of closing the door to the outside world whenever you need time to yourself. If you want to stay feeling young, however, don't isolate yourself for long periods. You need people.

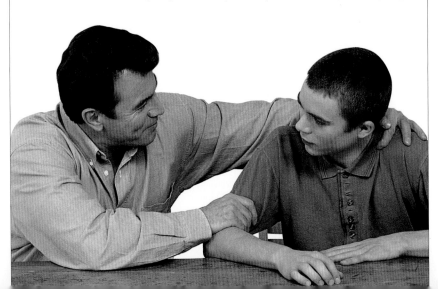

Time to kill?

Unemployed? Retired? According to research, people with too much time on their hands may soon feel bored, lonely, and worthless. Well, it doesn't take a genius to work that one out. Such negative feelings may lead to depression, introversion and, again, that 'old before your time' syndrome.

Enforced joblessness appears to hit men harder than it does women; men have a harder time adjusting and are less able to enjoy the rest or fill the gaps. With a positive attitude, however, life can become worthwhile and fulfilling again.

If newly work-free, the first thing to do is try to relax and enjoy the freedom of not having to get up and work every day. Of course, this may not be so easy if you have been made redundant from a job you enjoyed, or have money problems because of lack of work. However, a surprising number of people with more than adequate pension arrangements or finances still feel a strong sense of restlessness and bemoan the lack of purpose to their days without work.

Read the relaxation section overleaf. Years of hard work may have left you so stressed that you're probably much more wound up than you realize. It is not unreasonable to take two to three months just to unwind. Think about the times you may have gone on a two-week holiday, only to find that it wasn't until it was time to return home that you began to feel like relaxing. Now you have that time – make the most of it!

Your body-clock will gradually adjust to your new timetable and, when you are relaxed, you may find that all kinds of novel thoughts and ideas may appear in your brain. *Then*, and not until *then*, it is time to take stock of your life and begin to make some decisions about what you are going to do. This shouldn't be conscious 'time-filling', but merely deciding what *you* want out of life, what you can give – and going about it.

Start by using some of your time (plenty of it, in fact) thinking long and deep about yourself, and by exploring all the options.

Some questions to ask yourself are: Do I want to be creative? What can I do? Do I need further education? Do I need relaxing pursuits or stimulating pursuits? Do I want home-based activity or outside-home activity? Do I want to pursue ideas solo or with a group? Do I want physical or mental stimulation? Do I need to earn money? What do I have to offer others? Do close family need more of my time?

In many ways time is worth more than money, so use it, don't waste it – and certainly don't waste it feeling sorry for yourself.

Filling your life, not killing time

HOME-BASED IDEAS

❶ Books, CDs, correspondence courses for education either for pure pleasure or future profit.

❷ Write your own autobiography.

❸ Have a stab at that best-selling thriller or Booker prize winner.

❹ Create a new garden.

❺ Learn to cook.

❻ Get fit.

NON HOME-BASED IDEAS

❶ Join a Third Age Group.

❷ Get a part-time volunteer job with an organization whose work interests you.

❸ Utilize your talents with a local group e.g. you have a career in accountancy behind you, offer to keep the books for the drama group.

❹ Join the Ramblers Association.

❺ Get involved in community life, e.g. go to the local school and see what help they need.

❻ Start up a club yourself e.g. painting, photography, reading, walking.

RELAX AND RE-ENERGIZE

DO YOU FIND IT HARD TO UNWIND? ARE YOU OFTEN TIRED AND LACKING IN ENERGY, BOTH PHYSICALLY AND EMOTIONALLY? THESE MAY NOT SIMPLY BE NATURAL SIGNS OF INABILITY TO COPE WITH LIFE 'S PRESSURES AS YOU GET OLDER, BUT AVOIDABLE SYMPTOMS OF STRESS. THE NEXT FOUR PAGES WILL HELP YOU TO RELAX, RE-ENERGIZE AND CONTROL 'NEGATIVE STRESS' – SHEDDING THE YEARS AS YOU DO SO.

STRESS SIGNALS

STRESS OVERLOAD CHECKLIST

- Insomnia
- Irritability
- Loss of concentration
- Aches and pains for which no medical cause can be found
- Disorders of the digestive system
- Lack of libido
- Anxiety, panic, palpitations
- Dizziness or light-headedness
- Tiredness
- Muscle tension

'Stress' is the syndrome of the Millennium and billions of pounds are spent every year on trying to rid ourselves of it, and its symptoms – and even more money is wasted in time taken off work through 'stress-related illness'.

However, not *all* stress is bad. Many experts now believe that a certain amount of stress – with its increased production of adrenaline – is useful and, indeed, necessary for both personal and work-related survival, helping us to cope with tough workloads, react quickly to problems large and small, and so on. In this way it helps us, long term, to become more able, coping, stronger people, as each crisis is faced and beaten. Stress has even been shown to help increase IQ.

If we avoid stress-producing situations, the wisdom goes, it becomes harder and harder to deal with them. Our stress-tolerance levels 'shrink' and we become less adventurous and ever more likely to surround ourselves with everything that is familiar, unthreatening, undemanding. Back to the womb perhaps.

'Good stress' probably comes in short bursts, enabling you to cope with the demands of your own life and make some progress. If stress is not to harm you, it needs to be handled a bit like a 100-metre sprint or a hard session in the gym. You need recovery time, and the more stress you've been under, the more recovery you may need. It is lack of 'recovery time' or recovery strategies that creates 'bad stress' – and a selection of negative symptoms which are certainly not required.

Are you suffering from stress overload and lack of recovery? If you have more than one or two of the checklist of 10 symptoms (left), you probably are. Check it out now.

How best to deal with stress overload?

The first and obvious method is to look at the causes of your stress and try to reduce them to a manageable level. All the preceding pages offer advice on minimizing stress overload at work and at home. Section Five deals with sex problems.

Apart from this, the main strategy is to ensure that you get regular recovery periods and use a variety of methods to counteract the negative effects of stress, short-term and long-term. *This will include:*

● Practising short-term 'rescue methods' as instant – or semi-instant – ways to relieve stress after your own equivalent of the 100-metre sprint'. Regular use of these methods can help prevent long-term, more damaging health problems. (See overleaf.)

● Making time for recovery. This means regular periods of relaxation, both physical and mental, and doing all you can to ensure a good night's sleep (see overleaf and also see Self-indulgence on pages 130–31).

● If you have spare cash, you may also try relaxation therapies, such as aromatherapy (see page 129).

● Making time for exercise. Exercise is the modern form of 'fight or flight', and is one of the very best ways to ensure that negative stress symptoms don't build up. The exercise programmes in this book are ideal, combining aerobic work and strength with stretching. Stretching exercise is the cheapest form of therapy for tense muscles and general aches and pains. Aerobic and strength exercise rids you of surplus adrenaline and oxygenates the circulatory system, helping to prevent the symptoms of shallow, fast breathing as described on the right. Exercise is also good mental relaxation. (See Section Three for more information on what exercise to undertake.)

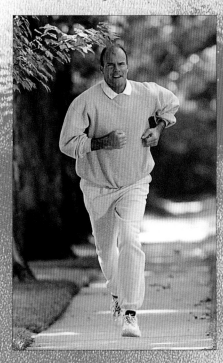

The long-term effects of stress overload

Long-term, too much stress can have a very real negative effect on your health. First you need to understand what happens when your body is under stress.

The hormones adrenaline and cortisol are pumped through the body to deal with every stressful situation. This is the age-old 'fight or flight' response which prepares the body to fight or run away. Symptoms of the raised levels of the hormones are fast-beating heart, tense muscles, sweating and, perhaps, fear. Breathing speeds up and becomes more shallow. The physical act of fighting, or running, reverts the hormones back to their normal levels and the symptoms of stress disappear.

These days, the fight or flight response is most likely to be produced in everyday situations, where fighting or running aren't an option, so the adrenaline is not dispersed and the stress symptoms remain and have a 'knock on' effect. For example, rapid breathing can lead to an imbalance of carbon dioxide and oxygen in the blood which can, in turn, lead to anxiety, palpitations and faintness or dizziness. If this continues, tiredness and muscle tension will also occur.

If stressful situations happen frequently and you don't take 'recovery steps' then there will be a harmful build up of the negative effects, which can lead to various health problems. Your immune system and circulation can be affected and long-term symptoms may include raised blood pressure, high cholesterol, depression, chronic insomnia and increased susceptibility to illness.

SHORT-TERM RESCUE METHODS
8 quick ways to relieve negative stress and tension

❶ Yawn. Opening the mouth wide and stretching out the jaw instigates a yawn which helps to relax the face, neck and lungs.

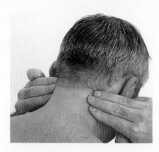

❷ Self-massage of the neck and shoulders. Sit in a chair, lower your head slightly so that back of neck elongates and, using your fingers on either side of your spine on the neck, exert medium pressure, moving the fingers slowly and firmly over the skin and up towards the lower skull. Find the knots of tension and massage for 2–3 minutes. Now bring your right arm across your chest and place your right hand on your left shoulder, making sure the shoulders aren't hunched up. Use the fingers of your right hand to massage the large muscle at the top of the shoulder firmly for 1 minute. Repeat to the other side.

❸ Self-massage of the face. Sit as relaxed as you can. Place the small fingers of both hands just above the inner eyebrows and use them to 'iron' the skin outwards towards the temples, fairly gently. Place the fingers on your cheekbones and use them to iron the skin upwards towards the forehead. Using the middle finger of each hand, gently massage the outer eye area (where 'crow's-feet' might be, if you had any!) and moving to the upper lid. Lastly, using the middle three fingers of each hand, massage all around your ears, starting at the lower back and working up the back and down the front.

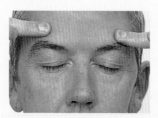

❹ Three-minute set of fairly gentle aerobic exercise, similar to a warm-up routine (see page 56). Try walking up and down stairs; marching on the spot; walking round the block.

❺ Long body stretch. Lie on the floor on your back, loosening any tight waistband. Place your arms on the floor above your head and stretch out your whole body as long as you can, breathing steadily throughout. Stay there for 3 minutes.

❻ Sitting stretch and shrug. Sit with the shoulders not hunched up, hands on your lap. Slowly shrug the shoulders up as high as they will go and back down, keeping your head still. Do this for 30 seconds. Now take your hands off your lap and bring your arms out to each side, down and backwards, with the fingers pointing towards the floor. Now bring them up until hands join above your head. Clasp fingers and pull your arms up to feel your chest and upper body stretching. Try to breathe steadily throughout. Relax.

❼ Sit in chair and shut your eyes. Place the palms of hands over the eyes. Relax your mouth. Visualize a peaceful and pleasing scene for you. Blue sea, blue skies, green fields, a big comfy bed – whatever. Concentrate on this image for as long as you can, breathing steadily.

❽ Deep breathing. Sit as relaxed as you can, hands on lap. Try to relax your abdomen, taking one deep, vocal breath as you do so (go 'ahhhh' on the out breath). Now sit for one minute, breathing more slowly and more deeply than usual, breathing in through the nose and out (with the 'ahhh' noise again) through the mouth. Do this several times a day. As you get more practice you should be able to breathe more deeply without feeling dizzy.

Making time for recovery

Periods of high stress should be balanced with similar periods of de-stressing. That is why it is important never to feel that such times are selfish or unnecessary. Here are some ideas on activities – and 'non-activities' – that may form your recovery periods.

● Any of the Self-indulgence ideas on pages 130–31, as long as they help you to feel relaxed rather than produce yet more stress.
● Hot bath with a good book.
● Good sex with someone familiar (sex with a new or demanding partner can increase stress levels).
● Relaxation audio tape/CD. Verbal tapes work for some. Special relaxation music or sound tapes/CDs can be helpful for many.
● Enjoyable meal, rich in complex carbohydrates (bread, rice, pasta, potatoes) and calcium (dairy produce), eaten in a relaxing place with enjoyable company.
● Period of undemanding, routine work, either at home or at work, e.g. catching up on your in-tray, catching up on research, sorting out your wardrobe.
● Sleep (see right).

WHAT NOT TO DO:
Don't resort to over-indulgence in alcohol, nicotine or drug-taking to relieve stress. Research shows that alcohol can increase depression, insomnia and actually increase stress levels long-term. Tobacco speeds up the ageing process and can kill. The research on soft drugs and stress is inconclusive, but the consensus is that reliance on any unnatural form of stress relief is counter-productive.

Beating insomnia

As we've seen, insomnia can be a direct result of stress overload (particularly anxiety) and if all the tips on these pages are followed, particularly those relating to exercise and relaxation, sleep quality should improve naturally. Conversely, however, as the body's ability to deal with stress can also be improved with a good night's sleep, we look at other possible causes of sleep problems and how to deal with them.

Your body needs sleep time to repair itself and to recover from the day's efforts. Adequate sleep helps regulate the ageing process, is the ultimate form of relaxation and, of course, energizes you by eliminating tiredness. If you can't sleep because you're stressed out, it becomes a vicious circle – with both the stress and the insomnia likely to get worse. First rule – deal with your stress following all the ideas on these pages.

The amount of sleep you need varies from person to person, but between 7–8 hours a night is considered average. The quality of this time spent in bed is important – shallow sleep from which you wake easily is not so refreshing as deep sleep and dream sleep.

Getting off to sleep: Have a familiar routine. Relax before you go to bed, physically and mentally. A non-demanding book or TV programme is ideal. Make sure you are warm (hot bath) and that the room is well aired and the bed and bedding comfortable. Eliminate noise and light (using earplugs/blackouts blinds/mask as appropriate). Think of enjoyable things.

Staying asleep: Waking in the night and being unable to get back to sleep is a common symptom of stress. This really is a case of having to eliminate the causes of the stress and anxiety and then the problem should take care of itself. To help break the pattern, herbal remedies containing valerian, hops or camomile, can be tried (available at all chemists and health-food shops).

These can be very effective and are non-habit-forming. You can also try to break the non-sleeping habit by going to bed later for a few nights, or by sleeping in another room. I wouldn't advise getting up, as this tends to confirm the habit rather than break it.

Disturbed sleep patterns due to jet lag can be helped with melatonin (available in the US). Too much alcohol can also cause mid-night waking and should be limited to 1–2 glasses in the evening maximum. Replace alcohol with a milk drink, which contains calcium and helps promote sleep.

Waking up refreshed: If you have a reasonable night's sleep but don't feel alert and 'raring to go' in the morning, consider these possible causes – too much alcohol last night? Lack of fresh air in the bedroom? Uncomfortable bed or sleeping position? Not enough sleep (go to bed earlier)? Some people are naturally less wide-awake in the mornings than others so, if you are feeling fine after half an hour or so and it's a normal pattern, it probably isn't anything to worry about.

TIRED ALL THE TIME

If you do sleep all right, but still tend to feel tired all the time, here are some possible reasons:
- Depression – linked to stress maybe. Seek help.
- Energy blocked. See energizing tips overleaf.
- Poor diet. Eat well, following the nutrition guidelines on pages 26–7 and making sure you include plenty of whole foods, iron-rich foods, and antioxidants.
- Lack of exercise. Exercise, far from tiring you out, is energizing.
- Boredom. If you've nothing exciting in life to look forward to, boredom is inevitable and often masquerades as tiredness.
- Lack of fresh air. Overheated and air-conditioned rooms at home and in the office can cause tiredness. Try to get out in the fresh air as much as possible.
- Stress – for explanation and remedies, see previous pages.

Re-energizing Yourself

Perhaps the best definition of youth is energy and vigour, which can be described as the physical and mental motivation and stamina to experience and enjoy life to the full.

Stress can be energizing in short bursts, as we've seen, but de-energizing if taken to overload. So, if you suspect that stress is sapping you of energy, take the appropriate steps to de-stress and relax as described on the previous pages and opposite.

You may wonder how you can be energized if you are relaxed – at first the two don't seem to go together – but when you are relaxed your 'energy channels', if you like, become unblocked. Think of your body as the fuel tank of a car. Stress is a tank full of low-quality, impure fuel. De-stressing is removing all the fuel from the tank and clearing it of impurities which may hinder performance. Once the tank is empty and clean it is now 'relaxed' and can be filled again with top-quality fuel – and suddenly you have 100% smooth and efficient performance.

We've dealt with the first two stages – here you learn how to fill the tank correctly.

Assessing your own energy levels

If you:
- are short on new ideas
- rarely make plans
- rarely do things on the spur of the moment
- rarely feel enthusiastic
- often feel under par, healthwise
- rarely feel clear-headed
- rarely feel optimistic
- often feel tired
– *you lack energy.*

To improve, first de-stress and relax as described earlier. Now concentrate on increasing energy-givers, and decreasing energy-takers. Here are some factors to look at:
● Improve diet. Energy robbers are *alcohol* (the worst thing you can indulge in if you lack energy), a junk-food diet (lacking in vitamins, minerals, antioxidants and phytochemicals),

highly refined carbohydrates such as white bread, pastries, biscuits, cakes (literally make you go to sleep). Energy-givers are good-quality highly nutritious foods as part of an overall balanced diet, including fresh fruit and vegetables, nuts, seeds, low-fat protein foods and complex carbohydrates, including plenty of vitamin B-rich foods and antioxidants. (For more information see page 27.)
● Improve exercise. As well as for basic stress relief, exercise is very useful in increasing energy levels. Most people think that exercise saps energy (you feel tired after a long walk, for example) but it oxygenates the body, increases circulation, increases brain power and increases muscle mass, all of which has an energy-enhancing effect long-term. It also helps you to sleep well.
● Breathe properly. If you are depressed or bored, as well as stressed or tense, you may not be breathing correctly. This will produce the effects listed on page 127 and has a direct result on your energy levels. Make a conscious effort to breathe properly all the time, and long-term try to improve your lifestyle so that you don't feel depressed or bored.
● Seek input. A too-safe life and/or boredom can lower energy levels. If you haven't done anything new or exciting for ages, make an effort to include something different in your life now and then. An exciting hobby or holiday, a challenge – see overleaf for ideas.
● Practical energy-blockers are life problems from which there seems to be no escape – e.g. a poor marriage, cramped living conditions, lack of money, unemployment, illness, leading to feelings of helplessness, hopelessness, depression, anger. Though you may be unable to solve the major problems in your life (i.e. you cannot remove the *cause*), it is still worth trying to remove the symptoms. Concentrate on clearing the fuel tank and hopefully energy levels will improve and the vicious circle can be broken.

Therapies may help to release your energy in these circumstances (see box right).

THERAPIES TO HELP UNBLOCK ENERGY

Reflexology: Foot massage, often done with the aid of essential oils. The feet are said to link up, through meridian lines, with all the body organs and when various spots on the feet are massaged the corresponding organ is 'tapped into' and toxins released. Reflexology is said to help release negative emotions too.

Power yoga: Classes are held combining yoga movements with aerobic movement – a powerful way to total relaxation and energy release.

Feng Shui: Re-organizing your home and/or work surroundings to make them more user-friendly and more energizing. Has been used in China for thousands of years and does seem to work.

T'ai Chi: Chinese preventive care – similar to yoga in some ways. Sequence of slow body movements practised regularly help to promote the flow of 'life energy' (*chi*).

Note: the therapies opposite will mostly also have an energizing effect, although principally used for relaxation. Similarly the therapies mentioned here will also have a relaxing effect.

THERAPIES FOR DE-STRESSING

If you have some spare cash, it may be worth considering trying therapy or classes to help reduce negative stress – and the effects of stress – long-term. Here are a few ideas:

YOGA: The oldest form of stress relief through exercise. Widely available and good for mental as well as physical stress. Inexpensive. Various different kinds, from basic no-frills yoga poses without the spiritual side, to much heavier stuff.

MEDITATION: Can be done in conjunction with yoga or as a therapy on its own. Once you have the hang of it, you can practise meditation at home or wherever you are, without outside help. Therefore also inexpensive. Can relax the body as well as the mind but, if you are very physically tense, best done in conjunction with relaxation exercise.

BREATHING CLASS: Few of us breathe properly; you can be taught how to do so, using diaphragm and abdomen correctly, by a practitioner. Can be taught in conjunction with other relaxation techniques.

RELAXATION CLASS: Should include breathing techniques, also may include 'tense and relax' exercises for the whole body, stretching, yoga.

MASSAGE: A regular professional massage can ease tension throughout the whole body and is particularly useful if you get tight painful neck, shoulder and back muscles – often stress-related. Different types of massage are available; try each until you find which you prefer.

AROMATHERAPY: Massage using calming essential oils is a good aid to relaxation and release of emotional and physical tension. See also Reflexology in the panel on the left.

Where to find them . . .
Your local library, the Internet, your local leisure or sports centre, your health-food shop, all will have details of therapies and classes available in your area.

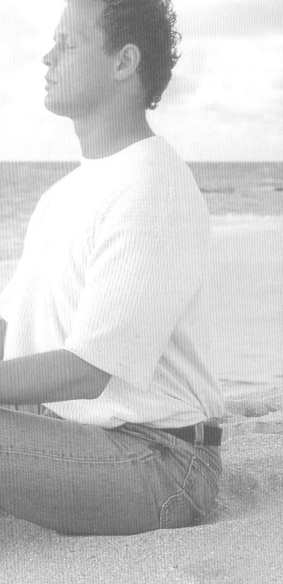

SELF-INDULGENCE

IT'S OFFICIAL – IT REALLY IS NO SIN TO TAKE TIME OUT TO ENJOY YOURSELF; MAKE TIME FOR YOU AND YOUR OWN NEEDS. ALL THE LATEST RESEARCH SHOWS THAT WE'RE MORE YOUTHFUL – AND LIVE LONGER AND HEALTHIER LIVES – IF WE PRACTISE REGULAR SELF-INDULGENCE. HERE ARE SOME IDEAS. . .

Making time for you

Apart from work, sleep and obligations, what do you do? Sadly, for many people, the answer is 'very little'. And yet in mid-life it is more important than ever to set aside time just for yourself. With regular daily 'self-time', stress levels can be reduced and health improved.

For men who have spent years doing nothing but working themselves to exhaustion at work and then at home, being selfish is a novel concept. Think of it as introducing balance into your life. The best way to begin is consciously to set aside a certain time every day (half an hour minimum) and use it how you will (plenty of ideas follow).

If anyone shows disapproval, state your case (that it is free health care and life insurance and, incidentally, your right!) and don't feel guilty.

Good times of day to consider using as 'self-time' are halfway through the day or in the last hour before going to bed.

As well as daily 'self-time', introduce weekly 'self-time' of at least 2–3 consecutive hours, and annual 'self-time' of at least two weeks. Try to spend some 'self-time' on who you want to be, as well as what you want to do – and spend at least some time doing absolutely nothing at all!

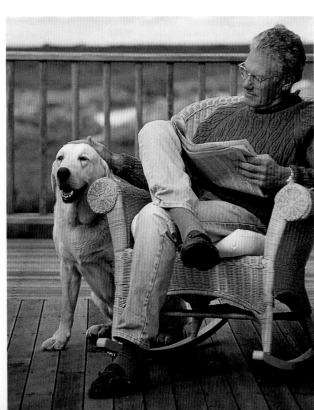

Who do you want to be?

During time for your self it is good to include some time on your self-potential. If, at age 40, 50, 60, you feel that much of your potential is exhausted, that is very ageing – and untrue. You may, realistically, not be in line for the Top Job or for making millions, but your Self is much greater than that. It is time to explore other areas of yourself and who you want to be. How about:

Increasing your charisma levels.
This whole book, I suppose, is about just that, but a lot of what makes charisma is self-belief. Spend some of your self-time affirming that you are sexy, clever, good-looking, loveable, personable, funny, successful . . . You may now be slim and fit and full of energy – but you just need that measure of self-confidence to make it all gel. Think positive.

Increasing your self-reliance.
This doesn't mean ignoring friends and opting for solitude – as we will see later, friends are very important. Neither does it mean being arrogant or stand-offish. But research shows that people are more popular with others if they exude a sense of being self-reliant rather than being dependent, needy, clingy.

Trying more positive thinking.
Research shows that people who 'look on the bright side' and talk in a positive manner are less likely to have coronary artery disease and more likely to have stronger immune systems than those who are negative. On a practical level, positive thought can effect the outcome of what you want. i.e. if you think it can happen – it probably will.

Increasing your brain power.
It is often said that as we age our brain power diminishes and thus our potential to use that brain. However, if you do regular brain workouts you can actually go on increasing your brain power – memory, concentration, intellect, speed, and so on – well into old age. Things that you do in your self-time will help to increase brain power, particularly new hobbies and challenges, and social interaction (see right). A stressed brain loses power, so following some of the anti-stress therapies (e.g. meditation, massage) discussed on page 129 will help you improve, as will exercise.

What do you want to do?

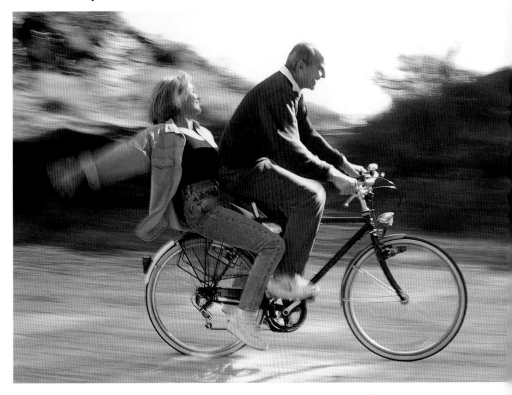

When you start out with 'self-time', you may think there is nothing you want to do with it. The best you can come up with is a glass of wine and a warm bath. Well, that's fine. In fact it's perfect. But when you get in the habit of self-time you will find that gradually you can think of hundreds of things you want to do.

Do what you want – as long as it's something you enjoy! Whether you have five minutes to look at a marvellous painting or three hours to indulge in the gourmet meal of a lifetime, enjoyment is good for you. Latest research shows that people who experience pleasure on a regular basis have a more efficient immune system than people who don't. It doesn't matter what the pleasure-factor is, as long as it is pleasurable for you. It could even be helping others – the feedback you get can really be a pleasure.

Fun and laughter: Laughter can reduce stress, reduce your blood pressure, heal minor ailments and improve general health. It is also pleasurable. Try to build light-heartedness and a good laugh into every day. A friend who makes you laugh is worth so much (see below). Failing that, your favourite TV comedian, a humorous book or even scouring your brain for funny memories can do the trick. As you go about your daily life, you should also keep your eyes, ears and brain open for the funny side of life. The observant mind is also more youthful than the closed mind!

Friends: Yet more research shows that people with a good circle of friends and/or family have reduced levels of stress and anxiety. For the purpose of self-indulgence, aim to see friends you feel comfortable and happy with rather than acquaintances who make you feel tense or inadequate. Phone friends regularly and use self-time to see them.

Hobbies and challenges: 'I haven't time for hobbies' is a typical male cry. Which is a shame, as all research indicates that hobbies keep the brain working well and keep you young. New ideas actually increase brain-power. Music

(playing or even listening) increases your power to reason and to carry out other tasks.

Challenges: Whether it is learning to rally drive, fly a helicopter or do the Rubik's cube – new challenges have a similar beneficial effect as well as increasing your self-confidence when successfully completed. Other challenges of an indoor nature could include writing a book, painting a master-piece or baking a cake. Anything can be a challenge if it is something that stretches you.

Holidays and travel: Choose holidays that you really will enjoy and if you have to have a family holiday where compromise is called for make sure to get a 'real' holiday of your own in which you do exactly as you want. This can be any type of holiday from an adventure (a challenge) to lying on the beach (doing nothing). Try to see something new as often as you can – travel, again, exercises the mind as well as increasing your pleasure factor. If you haven't

time for protracted holidays, even short one-day or overnight 'mini breaks' not far from home can be just as self-indulgent and fun. Use some 'self-time' to find out what's available.

Culture: How long since you went to the theatre or a concert, read a classic novel or went to a gallery? What interests you? What areas would you like to explore?

Nature: How long since you went for a really long walk, climbed a mountain, rode a horse, used your binoculars, paddled down a river, and so on? Nature is a healer, a calmer and awe-inspiring. It should be one of the huge pleasures of your life.

Nothing at all: Don't feel obliged to fill every minute of your 'self-time' being busy. If you are a busy person, there may be nothing better for you than to sit or lie, relax and do absolutely nothing. Maybe meditate a little, close your eyes and clear the mind.

It's your time – indulge yourself.

SPOT THE DIFFERENCE!

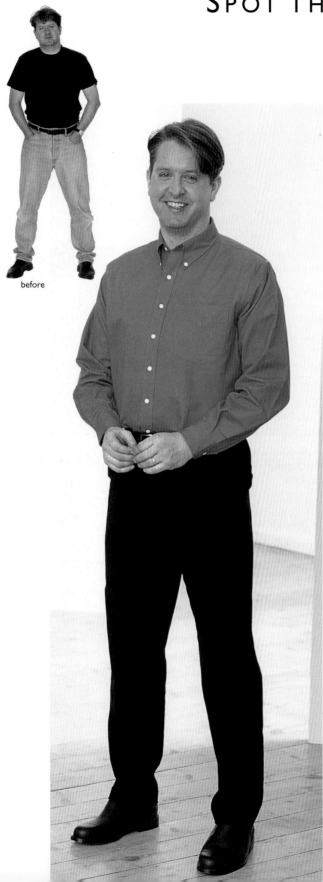

before

CHRIS DROPS 11 YEARS!

Chris Hampson went into the programme determined to succeed – and he did, achieving brilliant results both in his weight loss and waist circumference, reducing his body-fat percentage by over 2% and increasing his muscle mass by the same amount. He also increased his fitness in all areas, bettering his stamina by two whole levels and almost doubling the press-ups he could do.

His lifestyle has changed slightly – he is drinking a little less and aiming to fit more time for himself into his busy schedule. Everybody agrees that Chris does, indeed, look younger and the weight-loss suits his face *very* well. Says Chris, 'Healthier eating can fit into a normal lifestyle – I've proved it. I'm sure I'll have no trouble keeping the weight off now. I feel so much better too – weekend football is more enjoyable and I feel more confident about my future health.'

AFTER 10 WEEKS

Weight: 15 st 0 lb (95.45 kg)

Total weight loss: 1 st 2 lb (7.27 kg)

Chest: 43 in (1.07 m)

Hips: 42 in (1.05 m)

Body Mass Index: 28.7

Waist circumference: 36.5 in (91.25 cm)

Waist loss: 4 in (10 cm)

NEW FAT FORMULA SCORE: +2

Stamina (step test): Level 3

Strength: achieved 40 press-ups

Flexibility: achieved Level 4

Posture: passed the test

NEW FITNESS SCORE: -6

NEW HEALTH CHECK SCORE: -4

Total Score for all Assessments: -8

Actual age: 41

Real Age 10 weeks ago: 44

REAL AGE NOW: 33

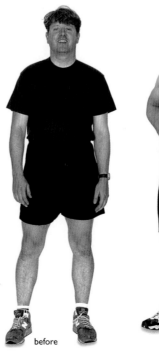

before

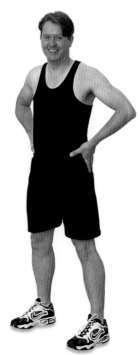

NOW CHECK OUT HOW THE FOUR PARTICIPANTS, ASSESSED AT THE START OF THE 10-WEEK PROGRAMME ON PAGES 8–9 AND 18–19, GOT ON. WE THINK THEY ALL DID INCREDIBLY WELL. THEY CERTAINLY LOOK TERRIFIC AND THEY ALL SAY THEY FEEL MUCH BETTER. IN TOTAL, THEY TOOK AN AMAZING 51 YEARS OFF THEIR REAL AGES!

CHRIS DROPS 14 YEARS!

AFTER 10 WEEKS

Weight: 12 st 12 lb (81.82 kg)

Total weight loss: 11 lb (5 kg)

Chest: 39.75 in (99.4 cm)

Hips: 41 in (1.03 cm)

Body Mass Index: 26.7

Waist circumference: 36 in (90 cm)

Waist loss: 3 in (7.5 cm)

NEW FAT FORMULA SCORE: +2

Stamina (step test): Level 3

Strength: achieved 21 press-ups

Flexibility: achieved Level 4

Posture: passed the test

NEW FITNESS SCORE: -5

NEW HEALTH CHECK SCORE: -4

Total Score for all the Assessments: -7

Actual age: 48

Real Age 10 weeks ago: 55

REAL AGE NOW: 41

before

In 10 weeks Chris Hall not only looks like a new man – he acts like one too! Much leaner, much fitter, with a more well-defined shape and more than 100% increase in his upper-body strength, Chris is proof that if you want to shed the years – you can.

He altered his body composition, shedding nearly 2.5% body fat and replacing it with nearly 2.5% lean muscle, and he managed to get rid of most of that gut in the 10 weeks. His BMI is almost down to the recommended level too.

To his 'new body' we added the final touches of a decent haircut, shedding *that* moustache and dressing him in some well-cut clothes – and the transformation was complete.

Says Chris, 'I found the whole thing surprisingly pleasant – the exercise was the hardest, but what kept me going was the benefits it brought – it's a subtle process, but I had a sense of a lighter mood, I feel more relaxed and also more alert. Several people have commented that I look younger and better.'

Chris hopes to lose a few more pounds in the months ahead and will continue with his exercise regime. 'I want go grow old not only gracefully, but healthily as well,' he says. 'And I'm determined to do so.'

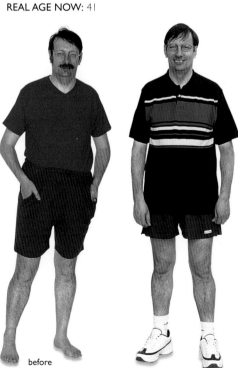

before

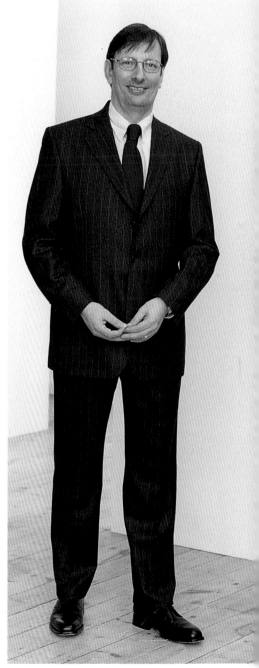

NOEL DROPS 15 YEARS!

Noel Ahearne was only a little overweight at the start of the programme and his six-pound loss brings his BMI virtually to the correct level. What really mattered was the phenomenal loss around his waist – four whole inches means that his 'pot belly' really is a thing of the past now. 'I'm so pleased about that,' says Noel. 'That was the one thing I really wanted to achieve, and I did. I hated my gut! All I did was cut out most of the junk food and cut back a bit on the alcohol.'

It was the exercise programme that helped Noel to achieve this, as well as increasing his flexibility by an amazing 350%, his stamina by one complete level and, although his strength didn't increase a lot, his posture improved 100%.

Noel cut back on smoking when he was able, though he found it difficult to cut back on both sweet treats and cigarettes at the same time. 'But I did find that when you are exercising aerobically you just can't smoke, so it did help me to cut down. I'm not going to let myself go again – I shall go to my local gym three times a week and pledge never to wear 38 inch-waist trousers again.'

before

AFTER 10 WEEKS

Weight: 12 st 3 lb (77.73 kg)

Total weight loss: 6 lb (2.7 kg)

Chest: 39.25 in (98.13 cm)

Hips: 38.5 in (95.38 cm)

Body Mass Index: 25.4

Waist circumference: 34 in (85 cm)

Waist loss: 4 in (10 cm)

NEW FAT FORMULA SCORE: -2

Stamina (step test): Level 3

Strength: achieved 21 press-ups

Flexibility: achieved Level 4

Posture: passed the test

NEW FITNESS SCORE: -5

NEW HEALTH CHECK SCORE: 0

Total Score for all Assessments: -7

Actual age: 51 (had birthday since start of programme)

Real Age 10 weeks ago: 59

REAL AGE NOW: 44

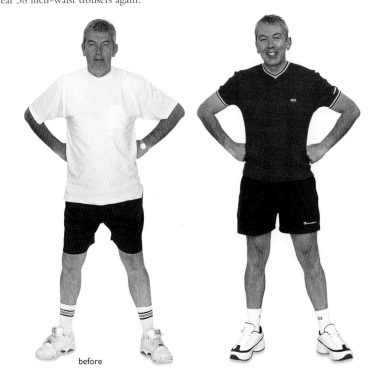

before

ROGER DROPS 11 YEARS!

AFTER 10 WEEKS

Weight: 14 st 1 lb (89.55 kg)

Total Weight Loss: 9 lb (4.1 kg)

Chest: 42 in (1.05 cm)

Hips: 38 in (95 cm)

Body Mass Index: 27.6

Waist Circumference: 36 in (90cm)

Waist loss: 3½ in (9cm)

NEW FAT FORMULA SCORE: +2

Stamina (step test): Level 2

Strength: achieved 17 press-ups

Flexibility: achieved Level 2

Posture: passed the test

NEW FITNESS SCORE: -2

NEW HEALTH CHECK SCORE: -2

Total Score for all Assessments: -2

Actual age: 52 (had birthday since start of programme)

Real Age 10 weeks ago: 61

REAL AGE NOW: 50

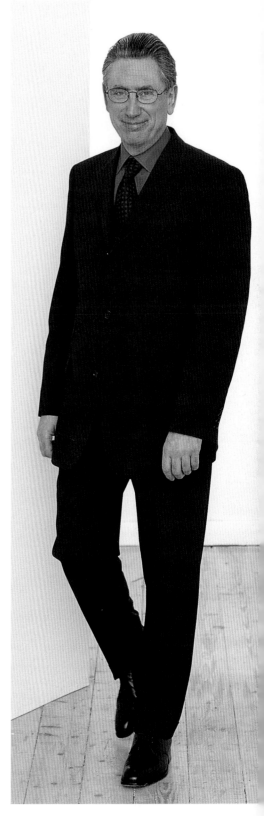

Roger Douglas freely admits that for the first few weeks of the exercise programme, he would sometimes feel physically sick from the exertion. 'But it soon wore off and by around about the middle of the programme I began to feel so much better. I remember going out to a party at the Dorchester and dancing most of the night – something I hadn't done for years! I seemed to have so much energy!'

Like the other participants, Roger improved tremendously in all areas of fitness. He beat all the others in the amount his stamina improved. In fact, his heart-rate during strenuous exercise decreased by a full 21 beats per minute – a sure sign of how well he did! Having scored very badly on the initial flexibility test, he has improved how far he can reach (on the sit-and-reach test) by 10 cm, moving himself up a whole category there, and noticeably reducing his general level of daily aches and pains. 'At last I find its easy to bend over to tie my shoe laces – something I couldn't even do ten weeks ago.'

He has made some lifestyle changes during the weeks and there are more in the pipeline to help reduce his stress levels – for instance, he has started getting the train to his new job instead of driving, and has just moved to the country to be nearer the office and his family.

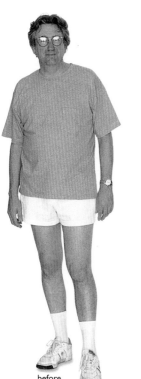

before

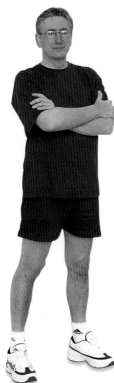

before

THE 10-WEEK PROGRAMME

To help you plan your 10 weeks, I have devised a weekly schedule which, if you follow it exactly, will mean by the end of the programme you will have covered all the areas you need to – diet, fitness, emotional health and well-being, and appearance, giving each enough time so that the plan really works.

The schedule works best for most people if Day One is a Monday, but it isn't imperative.

The first week is mainly concerned with familiarizing yourself with the programme and getting prepared – doing the Real Age Assessment, which is a crucial part of the plan, reading through the book, and acclimatizing to the fitness regime.

Subsequent weeks set out the programme in a logical sequence, giving you something to do on most days. Of course, the nutrition programme is continuous; once you've chosen your eating programme you follow it every day.

If, however, you prefer to organize your weekly programme in a slightly different way, then feel free to do so – but bear in mind the following guidelines:

● Home Circuits should be done a minimum of 3 times a week (4 if you like) and should be spaced out evenly throughout the week.

● Outdoor Exercise should be done a minimum of 3 times a week – most people would prefer to do this on alternate days to the Home Circuit, but it can be done on the same day if you like.

● Size and shape: we don't recommend that you keep hopping on and off the bathroom scales if weight-loss is one of your goals – a fortnightly weigh-in is adequate (if it helps motivate you). There are, however, spaces at the beginning and end of the programme to record your statistics.

YOUR STATISTICS NOW

Weight	
Chest	
Abdomen	
Waist	
Hips	
Body Mass Index *	
REAL AGE *	

see Assessments on pages 10–17

WEEK

day	activity
1	**Read through the entire book** and familiarize yourself with it. Get a full-length photo and head-shot taken of yourself.
2	Carry out **Assessments 1 and 2** *(see pages 10–13)*.
3	Carry out **Assessments 3 and 4** *(see pages 14–17)*. MY REAL AGE IS
4	Read page 24. Carry out **Food Preference Quiz** *(see pages 30–1)* and choose your eating programme. Shop for what you will need for the next 10 days (or as much as possible).
5	Start your **Home Circuit programme**, according to your REAL AGE *(begins on page 54 – see Chart on page 55 for further instructions)*. Use this session to familiarize yourself with the routine – allow yourself a longer time than normal.
6	Start **Outdoor Exercise Programme** *(see page 70)* according to your REAL AGE.
7	Do a **Home Circuit** session.

NOTES

● Depending upon the results of your Assessment 3 (Health Check), see what steps you can take to help yourself to better health apart from diet and exercise. Do you smoke? Begin to cut down. Do you drink more than the safe limits? Begin to cut down.

● Don't forget – if your health assessment results were poor, you must see a doctor as soon as possible to get a thorough professional check-up, and certainly before beginning any exercise.

WEEK 2

day	activity
1	Read through the **Sport for All** feature on pages 72–3 and see which sport possibilities attract you. See what facilities locally there are to carry out your chosen sport. Continue your prescribed **Outdoor Exercise** *(see pages 70–1)*.
2	Do your **Home Circuit** session *(see pages 54–67)*.
3	Do an **Outdoor Exercise** session.
4	Do a **Home Circuit** session.
5	Do an **Outdoor Exercise** session.
6	Do a **Home Circuit** session.
7	Decide on next week's menus and, if necessary, shop for the week ahead's food and drink. Have a go at your chosen sporting activity. *This is optional.* *Weigh yourself if you like.*

NOTES

● You'll need to give your new eating programme your full attention this week. Keeping a daily eating diary will help you to monitor what you eat and, if you need to lose weight and aren't losing around 4 pounds (2 kg) per fortnight you can look back at the diary and perhaps see where you were going wrong – with the nutritional help on pages 22–9.

● As I've said, you shouldn't weigh yourself too often, as weight does fluctuate and neither do we want to encourage you to be obsessive about your poundage. Also, we're concerned with body reshaping as much as fat loss. So if you need a regular incentive to keep going, you can measure your waist every week. See it shrink!

WEEK 3

day	activity
1	Do an **Outdoor Exercise** session *(see pages 70–1)*. Start looking after your skin *(see pages 82–3)*.
2	Do a **Home Circuit** session *(see pages 54–67)*.
3	Do an **Outdoor Exercise** session.
4	Do a **Home Circuit** session.
5	Do an **Outdoor Exercise** session.
6	Do a **Home Circuit** session.
7	Decide on menus for the following week and shop for food and drink, if necessary, or write list for anyone who may shop for you.

NOTES

● Don't forget, it is important to follow the correct Home Circuit and Outdoor Exercise sessions for your REAL AGE.

● Did you carry out the Assessments before beginning the programme?

● Have you read the chart on page 55 for Home Circuit instructions and read pages 70–71 for the Outdoor Exercise instructions? Exercising beyond your capabilities is dangerous. Exercising below your capabilities won't achieve results!!

WEEK 4

day	activity
1	Do **Outdoor Exercise** session *(see pages 70–1)*. Read through **Section Five** *(pages 94–107)*. Decide on areas that could be improved in your own sex life or relationships. **Make an action plan.**
2	Do **Home Circuit** session *(see pages 54–67)*.
3	Do **Outdoor Exercise** session.
4	Do **Home Circuit** session.
5	Do **Outdoor Exercise** session.
6	Do **Home Circuit** session.
7	Do **your chosen sporting activity** *(optional)*. Decide on next week's menus and, if necessary, shop for what you need. *Repeat* **all four Assessments**. If your REAL AGE has reduced, start doing **Home Circuit** and **Outdoor Exercise** according to your new REAL AGE *(see page 55 for Home Circuit chart and page 71 for your Outdoor Exercise instructions)*.

NOTES

● Don't forget that your eating programme and your skin care routine should now be regular fixtures in your life. Also, don't forget to work on points in your action plan for your sex life/relationships.

WEEK 5

day	activity
1	Do **Outdoor Exercise** session *(see pages 70–1)*. Do **Self Assessment** questionnaire on pages 110–11 in Section Six. Decide on goals and **read appropriate parts of Section Six.** Make action plan.
2	Do **Home Circuit** session *(see pages 54–67)*.
3	Do **Outdoor Exercise** session.
4	Do **Home Circuit** session.
5	Do **Outdoor Exercise** session.
6	Do **Home Circuit** session.
7	Do **chosen sport** *(optional)*. Decide on next week's menus and shop for food and drink.

NOTES

● Remember that to make real improvements in your fitness level you need to put real effort into what you are doing and increase the demands of your home circuits and outdoor activity every week (within your own capabilities). Results in exercise depend upon finding the balanced approach we call 'Sensible Sweating'. On the day that 16 press-ups become easy – you must do *more*!

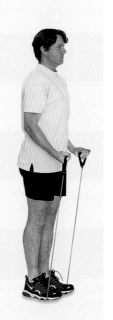

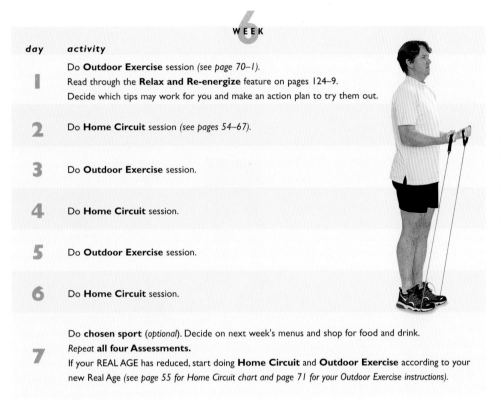

WEEK 6

day	activity
1	Do **Outdoor Exercise** session *(see page 70–1).* Read through the **Relax and Re-energize** feature on pages 124–9. Decide which tips may work for you and make an action plan to try them out.
2	Do **Home Circuit** session *(see pages 54–67).*
3	Do **Outdoor Exercise** session.
4	Do **Home Circuit** session.
5	Do **Outdoor Exercise** session.
6	Do **Home Circuit** session.
7	Do **chosen sport** *(optional)*. Decide on next week's menus and shop for food and drink. *Repeat* **all four Assessments.** If your REAL AGE has reduced, start doing **Home Circuit** and **Outdoor Exercise** according to your new Real Age *(see page 55 for Home Circuit chart and page 71 for your Outdoor Exercise instructions).*

NOTES

●Don't forget to work on ongoing health problems, such as cutting down on smoking and alcohol. Don't forget that your skincare programme and eating programme are ongoing. And are you still working on sex/relationships and relaxation and re-energizing techniques? All this will add up to how good you feel at the end of the programme.

WEEK 7

day	activity
1	Do **Outdoor Exercise** session *(see pages 70–1).* Book yourself a hairdressing appointment and, meanwhile, read pages 78–81 for some new ideas on how your hair could look. Make some decisions on what you're going to say to the hairdresser.
2	Do **Home Circuit** session *(see pages 54–67).*
3	Do **Outdoor Exercise** session.
4	Do **Home Circuit** session.
5	Do **Outdoor Exercise** session.
6	Do **Home Circuit** session.
7	Do **chosen sport** *(optional)*. Decide on next week's menus and shop for what you need.

NOTES

● Are you still working on areas of SELF that needed improvement? Work, financial and family problems can all add years and if you ignore problem areas they will affect the results of the programme. You need to make time to work on what you want and what you can give.

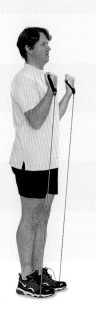

WEEK 8

day	activity
1	Do **Outdoor Exercise** session *(see pages 70–1)*. Read **pages 130–31** and decide whether you are under-indulging yourself! **Make an action plan** for fitting in more hedonistic time.
2	Do **Home Circuit** session *(see pages 54–67)*.
3	Do **Outdoor Exercise** session.
4	Do **Home Circuit** session.
5	Do **Outdoor Exercise** session.
6	Do **Home Circuit** session.
7	Do **chosen sport** (optional). Decide on next week's menus and shop for what you need. Do **Assessments** again and re-check your REAL AGE. If it has gone down, make sure next week to do correct **Home Circuit** and **Outdoor Exercise** sessions *(see page 55 for Home Circuit chart and see page 71 for Outdoor Exercise instructions)*.

NOTES

● Nearing the end of the programme, take some time to assess how you really feel now. Do you feel fitter? More energized? Slimmer? Stronger? Healthier? Are there areas of the programme that you've been neglecting? You still have two weeks to get those together.

WEEK 9

day	activity
1	Do **Outdoor Exercise** session (see pages 70–1). Read **style advice in Section Four** and look at the makeovers we did with our participants. Check out fashion brochures and the style ads in the men's magazines. Check out what's in the shops and note what you like. **Now go through your own wardrobe** and chuck out dated/useless/unflattering items or items that no longer fit you.
2	Do **Home Circuit** session (see pages 54–67).
3	Do **Outdoor Exercise** session.
4	Do **Home Circuit** session.
5	Do **Outdoor Exercise** session.
6	Do **Home Circuit** session.
7	Do **chosen sport** (optional). Decide on next week's menus and shop for what you need.

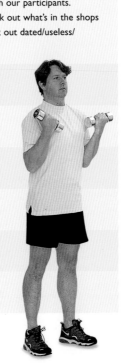

NOTES

● Still putting effort into your training and outdoor sessions? Still getting the sweat? You can improve as much as you want to improve. You know whether you're doing it. Do it!

10 WEEK

day	activity
1	Do **Outdoor Exercise** session *(see pages 70–1)*. Shop for new clothes, using all the knowledge and self-awareness you have gained. Get a photo of your new self taken.
2	Do **Home Circuit** session *(see pages 54–67)*.
3	Do **Outdoor Exercise** session.
4	Do **Home Circuit** session.
5	Do **Outdoor Exercise** session.
6	Do **Home Circuit** session.
7	Do **chosen sport** *(optional)*. *Repeat* **all four Assessments**. **Fill out new statistics** below, including your new age.

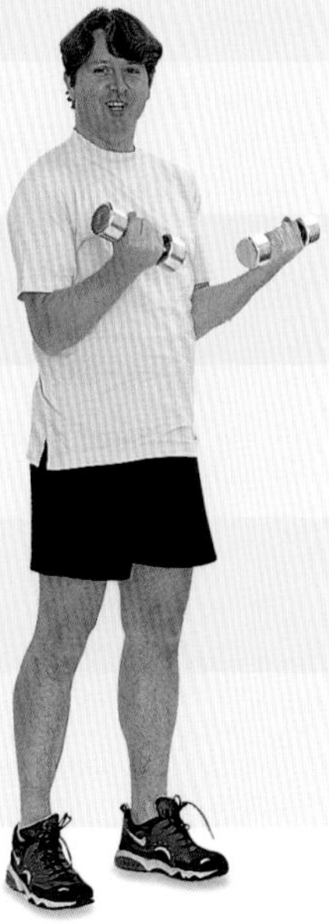

NOTES

● What now? If you need to lose more weight you can carry on with your eating programme as it is. If you are at your goal weight, increase portion sizes by a third.

● If you have yet to reduce your REAL AGE by 10 years you can continue with the exercise programme as laid out until you do. You can then follow the tips throughout the book for future body maintenance.

● Continue to work at areas of your life that have caused you stress in the past and always make sure to find time for yourself and your appearance.

YOUR STATISTICS AT END OF 10 WEEKS

Weight

Total Weight Loss

Chest

Abdomen

Waist

Hips

Body Mass Index*

REAL AGE *

(see Assessments pages 10–17)*

Congratulations on losing . . . . . . *years off your age in 10 weeks!*

Please write and let me know how you got on, and send me your 'before' and 'after' photos (with a stamped addressed envelope for their return) at the following address:

Judith Wills,
c/o Quadrille Publishing Ltd.,
Alhambra House,
27–31 Charing Cross Road,
London WC2H 0LS

The author would like to thank everyone at Quadrille, Lewis Esson, Mary Staples, Phillip Hodson, Rob Lander, Eddie Butler, Ceril Campbell, Michaejohn Hairdressing, Ian Hooton, Jane Turnbull and Tony Allen for their help and enthusiasm during the conception and production of this book.

Also many thanks to Chris Hampson, Chris Hall, Noel Ahearne and Roger Douglas for their dedicated participation in the 10–week programme.

THE PHOTOGRAPHS IN THIS BOOK WERE TAKEN SPECIALLY BY IAN HOOTON, EXCEPT THE FOLLOWING:

21 The Image Bank/Britt Erlanson; 53 Tony Stone Images/Gary Nolton; 70-71 Tony Stone Images/Bruce Ayres; 72-3 Corbis/Westlight © R W Jones; 77 The Image Bank/Britt Erlanson; 82-3 Tony Stone Images/Elie Bernager; 84-5 The Image Bank/Jaun Alvarez; 95 The Stock Market; 109 The Image Bank/Yellow Dog Productions; 12-13 Tony Stone Images/Greg Pease; 14 The Image Bank/Romilly Lockyer; 115 The Image Bank/David Vance; 116-17 Tony Stone Images/Bruce Ayres; 118 Explorer/Luria; 120 The Image Bank/Britt Erlanson; 121 Explorer/Rouchon; 122 Explorer/Rouchon; 122 The Stock Market/Ariel S Kelly; 123 Tony Stone Images/Lori Adamski Peek; 124-5 Tony Stone Images/I Burgman/P Boorman; 125 The Stock Market/Paul Barton; 127 The Image Bank/Patti McConville; 128-9 The Image Bank/Mori Kaz; 130 The Image Bank/White/Packert; 131 Tony Stone Images/Elie Bernager.

THE AUTHOR, THE PUBLISHER AND CERIL CAMPBELL WOULD LIKE TO THANK THE FOLLOWING FOR SUPPLYING ITEMS OF CLOTHING AND ACCESSORIES FOR PHOTOGRAPHY:

Adidas (tel 0161 419 2839)
Boss (tel 0171 589 5522)
Burton Menswear (tel 0171 291 2111)
Champion (tel 0181 840 7372)
Chipie (tel 0171 700 6470)
Debenhams (tel 0171 408 4444)
Dollond & Aitchison (tel 0121 706 6133)
Gap (tel 0800 427 789)
Hackett (tel 0171 738 8666)
Hanes (tel 0181 840 5505)
High & Mighty (tel 0171 723 8754)
John Lobb (tel 0171 930 3664)
Johnny Moke (tel 0171 351 2232)
Kelsey (tel 0171 404 1616)
Littlewoods Catalogue (tel 0345 888 222)
Marks & Spencer (tel 0171 935 4422)
Mulberry (tel 0171 491 3900)
Nike (tel 0800 056 1640)
Ozwald Boateng (tel 0171 734 6868)
Racing Green (tel 0113 238 2444)
Thomas Pink (tel 0171 498 3882)
Versace Classic V2 from Grattan Catalogue (tel 0345 444 333)

p 79 purple shirt Thomas Pink; p 80 blue button-down shirt Hackett; p 81 blue brushed cotton shirt Racing Green, white T-shirt Hanes; p 86 (top) navy moleskin jacket Boss, beige shirt Boss, grey trousers, Boss, belt Mulberry, brown suede loafers Johnny Moke; p 86 (bottom) brushed cotton blue check shirt Hackett, yellow rib cotton crew-neck sweater Hackett, navy needle-cord pleat trousers Hackett, brown deck shoes Timberland at Littlewoods Catalogue; p 87 (left) chalk-grey stripe suit Hackett, blue shirt Hackett, wine-coloured silk tie Hackett, black lace-up shoes Johnny Moke, glasses DKNY from Dollond & Aitchison; p 87 (right) all glasses from Dollond & Aitchison (2 Alain Mikli, 3 Armani, 4 DKNY, 5 Armani, 6 Silhouette); p 88 black moleskin jeans Racing Green, black jodhpur boots Littlewoods, grey striped wool sweater Burton Menswear; p 89 (left) blue/grey four-button suit Boss, airforce blue shirt Boss, airforce blue tie Boss, brogue shoes Johnny Moke; p 89 (centre) blue/grey four-button suit Boss, black two-button casual shirt Versace Classic V2 from Grattan Catalogue, leather belt Hackett, black buckle shoes Lobb; p 89 (right) Jacky Peer grey tracksuit High and Mighty, Ungaro purple Aertex sweatshirt High and Mighty, black puma lace-ups Littlewoods; p 90 100%-cashmere blazer Ozwald Boateng, white T-shirt Gap, relaxed-fit chinos Marks & Spencer, pleated brown leather belt Mulberry, brown suede loafers Johnny Moke; p 91 (left) Oxford button-down shirt Ralph Lauren at Littlewoods Catalogue, navy moleskin trousers Marks & Spencer, deck shoes Timberland at Littlewoods Catalogue, plaited brown leather belt Mulberry, navy wool sweater with collar Hackett; p 91 (right) black suit Boss, purple shirt and tie Boss, black lace-up shoes Johnny Moke; p 92 (centre) grey suit Boss, grey button-down shirt Racing Green, black lace-up shoes Johnny Moke, glasses Dollond and Aitchison; p 92 (right) tartan cotton shirt with cord collar Mulberry, camel moleskin trousers Mulberry, belt Mulberry, brown brogue shoes Johnny Moke; p 93 grey tweed jacket with blue windowpane check Hackett, pink cut-away collar shirt Hackett, pink and blue spot tie Hackett, grey flannel trousers Hackett, black brogue shoes Littlewoods; p 132 button-down blue shirt Hackett, black moleskin jeans Racing Green, black jodhpur boots Littlewoods; p 132 (right) Chris's own black T-shirt and shorts, trainers Nike; p 133 (bottom centre) navy-short-sleeved striped polo shirt Debenhams, blue sports shorts Hanes, white trainers Ellesse at Littlewoods, socks Adidas; p 133 (right) chalk-grey stripe suit Hackett, wine-coloured silk tie Hackett, button-down collar shirt Ralph Lauren at Littlewoods Catalogue, black lace-up shoes Johnny Moke, glasses DKNY from Dollond & Aitchison; p 134 (left) stripe suit, orange shirt and tie Kelsey, black lace-up shoes Johnny Moke; p 134 (right) red v-neck T-shirt Energie by Chipie, blue cotton jersey shorts Champion, white trainers Ellesse at Littlewoods; p 135 (centre) blue T-shirt 'Old Ireland' at Grattans Catalogue, navy shorts Nike, white trainers Ellesse at Littlewoods; p 135 (right) grey suit, shirt and tie Boss, black lace-up shoes Johnny Moke, glasses Dollond & Aitchison.

Please note that the clothing shown in the book may not all be available by the time of publication. There will, however, be similar items available in the credited outlets from the current season's collections by the same designers.